OTHER FAST FACTS BOOKS

Fast Facts for the NEW NURSE PRACTITIONER: What You Really Need to Know in a Nutshell, 2e (*Aktan*)

Fast Facts for the ER NURSE: Emergency Department Orientation in a Nutshell, 3e (*Buettner*)

Fast Facts About GI AND LIVER DISEASES FOR NURSES: What APRNs Need to Know in a Nutshell (*Chaney*)

Fast Facts for the MEDICAL–SURGICAL NURSE: Clinical Orientation in a Nutshell (*Ciocco*)

Fast Facts on COMBATING NURSE BULLYING, INCIVILITY, AND WORKPLACE VIOLENCE: What Nurses Need to Know in a Nutshell (*Ciocco*)

Fast Facts for the NURSE PRECEPTOR: Keys to Providing a Successful Preceptorship in a Nutshell (*Ciocco*)

Fast Facts for the OPERATING ROOM NURSE: An Orientation and Care Guide in a Nutshell (*Criscitelli*)

Fast Facts for the ANTEPARTUM AND POSTPARTUM NURSE: A Nursing Orientation and Care Guide in a Nutshell (*Davidson*)

Fast Facts for the NEONATAL NURSE: A Nursing Orientation and Care Guide in a Nutshell (*Davidson*)

Fast Facts About PRESSURE ULCER CARE FOR NURSES: How to Prevent, Detect, and Resolve Them in a Nutshell (*Dziedzic*)

Fast Facts for the GERONTOLOGY NURSE: A Nursing Care Guide in a Nutshell (*Eliopoulos*)

Fast Facts for the LONG-TERM CARE NURSE: What Nursing Home and Assisted Living Nurses Need to Know in a Nutshell (*Eliopoulos*)

Fast Facts for the CLINICAL NURSE MANAGER: Managing a Changing Workplace in a Nutshell, 2e (*Fry*)

Fast Facts for EVIDENCE-BASED PRACTICE: Implementing EBP in a Nutshell, 2e (*Godshall*)

Fast Facts for Nurses About HOME INFUSION THERAPY: The Expert's Best Practice Guide in a Nutshell (*Gorski*)

Fast Facts About NURSING AND THE LAW: Law for Nurses in a Nutshell (*Grant, Ballard*)

Fast Facts for the L&D NURSE: Labor & Delivery Orientation in a Nutshell, 2e (*Groll*)

Fast Facts for the RADIOLOGY NURSE: An Orientation and Nursing Care Guide in a Nutshell (*Grossman*)

Fast Facts on ADOLESCENT HEALTH ... **:** A Care Guide in a Nutshell (*Herrman*)

Fast Facts for the FAITH COMMUNIT... Nutshell (*Hickman*)

Fast Facts for the CARDIAC SURGERY ... Nutshell, 2e (*Hodge*)

Fast Facts About the NURSING PROFESSION: Historical Perspectives in a Nutshell (*Hunt*)

Fast Facts for the CLINICAL NURSING INSTRUCTOR: Clinical Teaching in a Nutshell, 2e (*Kan, Stabler-Haas*)

Fast Facts for the WOUND CARE NURSE: Practical Wound Management in a Nutshell (*Kifer*)

Fast Facts About EKGs FOR NURSES: The Rules of Identifying EKGs in a Nutshell (*Landrum*)

Fast Facts for the CRITICAL CARE NURSE: Critical Care Nursing in a Nutshell (*Landrum*)

Fast Facts for the TRAVEL NURSE: Travel Nursing in a Nutshell (*Landrum*)

Fast Facts for the SCHOOL NURSE: School Nursing in a Nutshell, 2e (*Loschiavo*)

Fast Facts About CURRICULUM DEVELOPMENT IN NURSING: How to Develop & Evaluate Educational Programs in a Nutshell (*McCoy, Anema*)

Fast Facts for DEMENTIA CARE: What Nurses Need to Know in a Nutshell (*Miller*)

Fast Facts for HEALTH PROMOTION IN NURSING: Promoting Wellness in a Nutshell (*Miller*)

Fast Facts for STROKE CARE NURSING: An Expert Guide in a Nutshell (*Morrison*)

Fast Facts for the MEDICAL OFFICE NURSE: What You Really Need to Know in a Nutshell (*Richmeier*)

Fast Facts for the PEDIATRIC NURSE: An Orientation Guide in a Nutshell (*Rupert, Young*)

Fast Facts About the GYNECOLOGICAL EXAM FOR NURSE PRACTITIONERS: Conducting the GYN Exam in a Nutshell (*Secor, Fantasia*)

Fast Facts for the STUDENT NURSE: Nursing Student Success in a Nutshell (*Stabler-Haas*)

Fast Facts for CAREER SUCCESS IN NURSING: Making the Most of Mentoring in a Nutshell (*Vance*)

Fast Facts for the TRIAGE NURSE: An Orientation and Care Guide in a Nutshell (*Visser, Montejano, Grossman*)

Fast Facts for DEVELOPING A NURSING ACADEMIC PORTFOLIO: What You Really Need to Know in a Nutshell (*Wittmann-Price*)

Fast Facts for the HOSPICE NURSE: A Concise Guide to End-of-Life Care (*Wright*)

Fast Facts for the CLASSROOM NURSING INSTRUCTOR: Classroom Teaching in a Nutshell (*Yoder-Wise, Kowalski*)

Forthcoming FAST FACTS Books

Fast Facts About PTSD: A Guide for Nurses and Other Health Care Professionals (*Adams*)

Fast Facts for the OPERATING ROOM NURSE: An Orientation and Care Guide in a Nutshell, 2e (*Criscitelli*)

Fast Facts for TESTING AND EVALUATION IN NURSING: Teaching Skills in a Nutshell (*Dusaj*)

Fast Facts for the CLINICAL NURSING INSTRUCTOR: Clinical Teaching in a Nutshell, 3e (*Kan, Stabler-Haas*)

Fast Facts for the CRITICAL CARE NURSE: Critical Care Nursing in a Nutshell, 2e (*Landrum*)

Fast Facts for MANAGING PATIENTS WITH A PSYCHIATRIC DISORDER: What RNs, NPs, and New Psych Nurses Need to Know (*Marshall*)

Fast Facts About CURRICULUM DEVELOPMENT IN NURSING: How to Develop & Evaluate Educational Programs in a Nutshell, 2E (*McCoy, Anema*)

Fast Facts About the GYNECOLOGIC EXAM: A Professional Guide for NPs, PAs, and Midwives, 2e (*Secor, Fantasia*)

FAST FACTS on
COMBATING NURSE BULLYING, INCIVILITY, and WORKPLACE VIOLENCE

Maggie Ciocco, MS, RN, BC, is currently a nursing program advisor for the W. Cary Edwards School of Nursing at Thomas Edison State University, Trenton, New Jersey. She has more than 25 years of experience in nursing education, as a preceptor, mentor, staff development instructor, orientation coordinator, nursing lab instructor, and clinical instructor. Ms. Ciocco received her master of science degree in nursing from Syracuse University; her bachelor of science degree in nursing from Seton Hall University, South Orange, New Jersey; and her associate degree from Ocean County College, Toms River, New Jersey. She has been an American Nurses Credentialing Center board-certified medical–surgical nurse for more than 20 years. Throughout her years as an educator, she has established preceptorship programs in acute, subacute, and long-term care settings. She is a member of the National League for Nursing and Sigma Theta Tau. Ms. Ciocco was awarded the Sigma Theta Tau–Lambda Delta Chapter Hannelore Sweetwood Mentor of the Year award in 2012. She is the author of *Fast Facts for the Medical–Surgical Nurse: Clinical Orientation in a Nutshell* and *Fast Facts for the Nurse Preceptor: Keys to Providing a Successful Orientation in a Nutshell.*

FAST FACTS on COMBATING NURSE BULLYING, INCIVILITY, and WORKPLACE VIOLENCE

What Nurses Need to Know in a Nutshell

Maggie Ciocco, MS, RN, BC

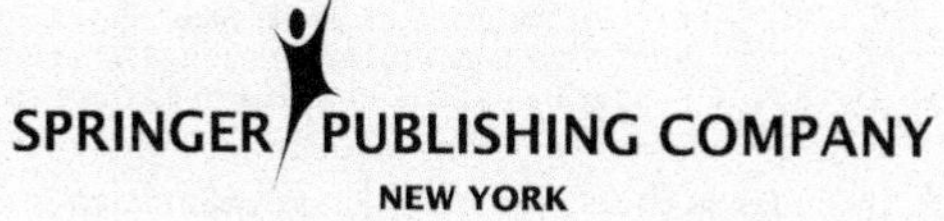
SPRINGER PUBLISHING COMPANY
NEW YORK

Springer Publishing Company, LLC
11 West 42nd Street
New York, NY 10036
www.springerpub.com

Acquisitions Editor: Elizabeth Nieginski
Senior Production Editor: Kris Parrish
Compositor: Westchester Publishing Services

ISBN: 978-0-8261-3817-0
e-book ISBN: 978-0-8261-3818-7

17 18 19 20 / 5 4 3 2 1

Library of Congress Cataloging-in-Publication Data

Names: Ciocco, Margaret Curry, author.
Title: Fast facts on combating nurse bullying, incivility, and workplace violence : what nurses need to know in a nutshell / Maggie Ciocco.
Other titles: Fast facts (Springer Publishing Company)
Description: New York, NY : Springer Publishing Company, LLC, [2017] | Series: Fast facts | Includes bibliographical references and index.
Identifiers: LCCN 2017013469| ISBN 9780826138170 (hard copy : alk. paper) | ISBN 9780826138187 (ebook)
Subjects: | MESH: Nurses—psychology | Bullying—prevention & control | Students, Nursing—psychology | Interprofessional Relations | Workplace Violence—prevention & control | Nurses' Instruction
Classification: LCC RT1 | NLM WY 88 | DDC 610.730601—dc23
LC record available at https://lccn.loc.gov/2017013469

Printed in the United States of America by Gasch Printing.

To the "Other Ones" —

My previous books were dedicated to fellow nursing professionals and educators who made me the nurse I am today. I was educated by some of the best nursing professors and instructors in the profession, and I became a nurse educator because of them. I will never forget their kindness, strength, and advocacy for their patients and students. What they taught me was invaluable. But then there were the "other ones." These other nurses also taught me, and their example influenced me as well, perhaps even to a greater extent.

I began my career as does every other student nurse, with the naïve impression that nursing is a profession filled with wondrous, gentle souls living out a vocation of service to humanity. The nurses who epitomized these qualities treated all that they encountered with gentleness and compassion. I vowed that someday, I would be "just like them" and endeavored to model their behavior. But I also observed the "other ones"—those other nurses I have encountered throughout my career. I listened when they spoke to each other and I observed how, as instructors, they interacted with students. I gathered remembrances of tears, whispered rumors, sneered accusations, and criticisms. I collected feelings of being ignored, rebuffed, and mocked. I witnessed the example of every clinical instructor who mistreated a student, every nursing professor who chose to "make an example" of a student's failing, every charge nurse who belittled a novice nurse in front of staff, every unit manager who disregarded a new employee, and the staff nurses who were snubbed, overlooked, or mistreated by each other and by nursing administration.

The lessons the "other ones" taught me were valuable as well. They taught me to endeavor to treat each nurse, no matter each one's time in the role, as a professional whose goal was similar to mine; to provide the best care each one could to a patient; and to offer the best education to a student. I would welcome each new nurse to the field and model the behavior of how we should treat each other. Today, I still meet some of the "best and brightest" this profession has to offer and it continuously renews my spirit and love of nursing. I also still meet the "other ones" as well, and I continue to learn.

A special thank-you to Filomela (Phyllis) Marshall, EdD, RN, CNE—Dean, W. Cary Edwards School of Nursing at Thomas Edison State University, Trenton, New Jersey—quite literally, the best boss I've ever had! You lead from the front, support from the back, and always walk alongside.

Thank you to Sarah Hopkins, for all your hard work and support. You have chosen the best job in the world . . . good luck always!

And finally, to the Dream Team.

Keep away from people who try to belittle your ambitions. Small people always do that. But the really great make you feel that you, too, can become great.

—Mark Twain

If I've learned anything from life, it's that sometimes, the darkest times can bring us to the brightest places and that our most painful struggles can grant us the most necessary growth.

—Danielle Koepke

Contents

Contributors *xiii*
Foreword Filomela A. (Phyllis) Marshall, EdD, RN, CNE *xv*
Preface *xvii*

1. **Bullying, Incivility, and Workplace Violence in Nursing: The Scope and Impact of the Problem** 1
2. **What Is a Bully?** 9
3. **Incivility in Nursing** 17
   Latoya N. Rawlins
4. **Bullying in Nursing** 29
5. **Understanding Workplace Violence in Health Care** 43
6. **The Cost of Nurse Bullying on the Health Care System** 57
7. **Bullying and the Nurse: Effects, Resolution, and Healing** 65
8. **The Responsibilities of Nursing Leadership and the Employer** 79
9. **Resisting a Bully** 89
10. **Nurse Bullying and the Law** 101
    Jackeline Biddle Shuler
11. **Bullying and the Student Nurse** 113
12. **Case Studies: Bullying and the Student Nurse** 125
13. **Bullying and the Novice Nurse** 137
14. **Case Studies: Bullying and the Novice Nurse** 143
15. **Bullying in Nursing Education** 153

16. Case Studies: Bullying in Nursing Education **163**

17. Case Studies: Bullying in Nursing Administration **173**

Bibliography *183*
Index *187*

Contributors

Latoya N. Rawlins, DNP, RN-BC
Clinical Assistant Professor of Nursing
Rutgers University
New Brunswick, New Jersey

Jackeline Biddle Shuler, JD, DNP, RN, CNE
Associate Dean of Faculty
Chamberlain College of Nursing
North Brunswick, New Jersey

Foreword

What mental images come to mind when you hear the word "bully"? Often it is the larger-than-life character looming over the small vulnerable person. It invokes an image of someone who is mean, hostile, and to be feared. How can that word be used in the same sentence as "nurse"? The image of the nurse is most usually associated with caring for, compassion toward, and healing of those who are sick and vulnerable.

Nurses have been rated by most Americans in the Gallup Poll for the past 15 years as the profession highest in honesty and ethics. How can a profession so trusted by the public be associated with bullying and incivility?

Incivility, bullying, and workplace violence in nursing are significant problems—so much so that the American Nurses Association (ANA) developed a position statement in 2015 addressing the issue (ANA, 2015). ANA's *Code of Ethics for Nurses With Interpretive Statements* notes that nurses are required to "create an ethical environment and culture of civility and kindness, treating colleagues, coworkers, employees, students, and others with dignity and respect" (ANA, 2015, p. 4). How is it that we find ourselves at this juncture?

This book explores the topic and gives the reader practical hands-on skills on how to identify and deal with this phenomenon.

It provides detailed information, emphasizing why it is not okay to put new nurses "through the wringer" because we were once in that position. It is not okay to undermine coworkers or discourage students' confidence. These tactics do not make us stronger. Bullying demoralizes us and sends exceptional young people with immense potential running from our profession. Now is the time for us to act. With the looming shortage in nursing, we must attract young, vibrant, caring, and creative individuals into nursing. We must nurture their spirit and keep them safe. Nursing must no longer tolerate this conduct.

Maggie Ciocco, the author, experienced this ugly behavior firsthand. Arriving at this institution wounded, she has, with the support of her coworkers, been able to accomplish so many positive things. With confidence restored, she is truly an advocate for all her students and those who work in the school of nursing. Well done, Maggie.

Filomela A. (Phyllis) Marshall, EdD, RN, CNE
Dean, W. Cary Edwards School of Nursing
Thomas Edison State University
Trenton, New Jersey

Reference

American Nurses Association. (2015). *Incivility, bullying, and workplace violence*. Retrieved from http://www.nursingworld.org/MainMenuCategories/WorkplaceSafety/Healthy-Nurse/bullyingworkplaceviolence/Incivility-Bullying-and-Workplace-Violence.html

Preface

In 1986, Judith Meissner wrote an article titled "Nurses: Are We Eating Our Young?" The article addressed how more experienced nurses often bullied new graduates and, instead of welcoming them to the profession, made their lives and work environment miserable. At the time of the writing, the article sent a shockwave throughout the profession of nursing. It was met with doubt on the surface because bullying and incivility in nursing had always been regarded as "our dirty little secret," but it succeeded in opening a dialogue among nursing professionals at all levels.

The original article has been referenced literally hundreds of times and the phrase "eating our young" was added to the popular lexicon. Many subsequent articles and books have been written and research studies conducted regarding how nurses of all ages and experiences treat each other in the workplace and in schools of nursing, and theories have been developed elaborating what leads to such behavior. Human resources departments in countless health care facilities have developed policies to deal with "lateral and vertical hostility" (bullying), incivility, and workplace violence. Schools of nursing now provide courses on ethics and fair treatment of colleagues. However, despite courses, human resources policies, employer reprimands, and employee punishments, the behavior of nurses toward each other has not improved.

So prevalent is the behavior that it is now felt that nurses have become desensitized. Very telling is the perspective shared by a third-year nursing student, who stated, "that was *your* generation; nurses don't bully anymore." She then reviewed current research and observed her fellow students and how they treat each other and nursing faculty and, in turn, are treated by hospital nursing and medical staff and clinical instructors. Upon reflection, she realized that the behavior is so common it is thought to be "normal" and part of the job or the initiation onto a new unit.

This text is intended to be a "field guide" to bullying and incivility: how to define, recognize, and deal with the behavior. It is not a text about fixing the profession of nursing so that nurses are uniformly supportive of each other and treat each other with kindness. Bullying and incivility will not be eliminated after reading an article or book. They *will* be eliminated when hospital and nursing administration, deans in academia, and professors of nursing recognize the problem, take seriously the complaints of the victims, successfully punish the perpetrators, screen for its presence prior to employment and school of nursing entrance, and educate all in how to recognize the problem and know how to assertively address the situation without hiding in fear. Bullying and incivility will be stopped when they are no longer tolerated!

Maggie Ciocco

1

Bullying, Incivility, and Workplace Violence in Nursing: The Scope and Impact of the Problem

In April 2015, the American Nurses Association (ANA) published a draft of its position statement on incivility, bullying, and workplace violence. It sought public comment on the document and its contents, and the final position paper was published later that year. The purpose of the statement was to convey the ANA's position that both nurses and their employers share a legal and ethical responsibility to establish and maintain a workplace that is free from incivility, bullying, and workplace violence. A work environment that is free from the psychological burden and financial instability caused by bullying is healthier for the entire team and, most importantly, for patients and their families.

After reading this chapter, the reader will be able to:

- List the provisions in the ANA *Code of Ethics for Nurses With Interpretive Statements* that deal with bullying
- List the three elements that form a "constellation of harmful events"
- Explain how bullying and incivility are unethical
- Explain why zero tolerance in bullying may not be effective
- Explain how bullying and incivility are considered an impairment like drug abuse

THE BOTTOM LINE

". . . the nursing profession will no longer tolerate violence of any kind from any source" (ANA, 2015a, p. 1). Why begin a book with a concluding sentence—with the bottom line? Why begin anything with the final thought? Because after generations of bullying in nursing, a major voice of nursing has published a definitive stance against the phenomenon. Because of violence in nursing for decades, someone in a position of power has finally said "enough." But will it be enough?

Fast Facts in a Nutshell

In a 1909 article published in the *New York Times*, Dr. Leon Harris noted that in the hospital in which he worked, there were multiple examples of nurses being bullied. He noted that "head nurses abuse their position of power" (Gaffney, DeMarco, Hofmeyer, Vessey, & Budin, 2012, p. 1) and that bullying "threatens to affect the welfare of hospital patients" (Castronovo, Pullizzi, & Evans, 2016, p. 210).

A GLOBAL PHENOMENON

The phenomenon of bullying in nursing is global, affecting every country on Earth. It is not isolated to the United States or to one particular specialty of nursing. Unfortunately, in many cultures, including our own, bullying has become accepted as "normal" behavior. "For nearly a century, some form of incivility, bullying, or violence has touched far too many members of the nursing profession. They affect every nursing specialty, occur in virtually every practice and academic setting, and extend into every educational and organizational level of nursing" (ANA, 2015a, p. 1). There are some studies indicating bullying is a global phenomenon:

- A British survey of more than 1,000 health care workers found that 44% of nurses had experienced "peer bullying" in the past year (Ariza-Montez, Muniz, Montero-Simó, & Araque-Padilla, 2013).
- A study of 5,000 hospital workers in Finland found that 5% of them had been bullied. Fifty percent of this group was nurses.
- In 2008, 511 nurses in Massachusetts stated that 21% of them had been bullied while at the same time 31% met the criteria for being bullies themselves.
- In 2006, a study among 4,000 critical care nurses in the United States found that 18% had experienced verbal abuse from another nurse. This same study revealed that these nurses rated the quality of communication and teamwork with other RNs as "fair or poor."
- Five hundred newly graduated nurses in New Zealand stated that "covert interpersonal conflict was common" (Dellasega, 2009, p. 52).
- Fifty-nine percent of nurses in Great Britain identified their nurse manager as a bully.
- Male and female nurses are affected alike, although female nurses are more likely found to be the perpetrators.

- More men (62%) are bullies and women are the most frequent targets of bullies (58%). Women bullies target other women (80%; Heathfield, 2016).

"A CONSTELLATION OF HARMFUL ACTIONS"

The ANA has stated that bullying, incivility, and workplace violence is part of a multifaceted problem of overt actions (and inactions) and covert activities that it states are a "constellation of harmful actions" (ANA, 2015a, p. 2). The side effects of this phenomenon not only ruin nursing relationships and unspoken trust with society, but also harm patients. The ANA urges nurses to acknowledge and recognize the different forms of aggression and focus their understanding and experience on eliminating it from the workplace.

The ANA defines "incivility" as any action that takes the "form of rude and discourteous actions, or gossiping and spreading rumors and of refusing to assist a coworker (ANA, 2015a, p. 2). Incivility, if left unchecked, can progress into bullying. Bullying can take many different forms including, as stated in the ANA position statement, workplace mobbing or the "adult" form of bullying. The third type of bullying, which leads to harmful action, stated by the ANA, is workplace violence. "Workplace violence consists of physically and psychologically damaging actions that occur in the workplace or while on duty" (ANA, 2015a, p. 4). It is endemic, meaning that it occurs in certain settings within health care such as the emergency department and psychiatric facilities, among others. It has been found that workplace violence like other forms of bullying is expected and is felt to be the norm in the profession of nursing. Health care leaders are seen to value the lives and well-being of patients over that of their staff.

MANY VOICES, ONE THOUGHT

As stated, the ANA as well as The Joint Commission and other international and national nursing specialty organizations have spoken out on bullying, incivility, and workplace violence in health care. Their statements include the following:

- "... inherent in accountability is responsibility for individual actions and behaviors, including civility. In order to demonstrate professionalism, civility must be present. . . . In professional practice, altruism is reflected by the nurse's concern and advocacy for the welfare of patients, other nurses, and other healthcare providers. . . . In professional practice, concern for human dignity is reflected when the nurse values and respects all patients and colleagues . . ." (American Association of Colleges of Nursing, 2008, pp. 23–24).
- "The nurse creates an ethical environment and culture of civility and kindness, treating colleagues, coworkers, employees, students, and others with dignity and respect. This standard of conduct includes an affirmative duty to act to prevent harm. Disregard for the effects of one's actions on others, bullying, harassment, intimidation, manipulation, threats or violence are always morally unacceptable behaviors" (ANA *Code of Ethics for Nurses* Provision 1.5, 2015b).
- The Joint Commission stated in the 2008 Sentinel Alert, "... organizations that fail to address unprofessional behavior through formal systems are indirectly promoting it and in 2009, The Joint Commission began requiring that organizations establish a code of conduct that defines and distinguishes acceptable and unacceptable behaviors to maintain their accreditation" (Larson, 2013).
- "Standards to make a zero tolerance policy work were developed by the American Association of Critical Care Nurses in 2004. . . . The six standards are authentic leadership, skilled communication, true collaboration, effective decision making, appropriate staffing that matches patient needs and competencies, and meaningful recognition" (Lachman, 2015, p. 41).
- "Intimidating and disruptive behaviors can foster medical errors, contribute to poor patient satisfaction and to

preventable adverse outcomes, increase the cost of care, and case qualified clinicians . . . to seek new positions (The Joint Commission, 2008)."

The ANA *Code of Ethics for Nurses* is the nursing profession's "non-negotiable ethical standard" (Lachman, 2015, p. 2). It is notable that the first four provisions outline what the ANA feels are the "essential values and commitments of the nurse, with four interpretive statements that are relevant to ethical issues surrounding disruptive behaviors" (Lachman, 2015, p. 39).

- **Provision 1.5: Relationships With Colleagues and Others**—Conveys that nurses must respect and be compassionate and caring toward all individuals with whom they interact, including colleagues and patients. Nurses should adhere to an obligation that all should be treated fairly with allowance of compromise and conflict resolution. This first statement excludes any forms of harassment or intimidating behavior. "Clearly, statement 1.5 strictly prohibits nurses from engaging in incivility, bullying or horizontal/lateral violence" (Lachman, 2015, p. 39).
- **Provision 2.3: Collaboration**—States that nurses should work collaboratively on a multidisciplinary team. In order for the team to be effective, each member must be able to trust and respect other members. The ability to share information and freely participate in mutual decisions regarding patient care is imperative. "Disruptive behaviors interfere significantly with nurses' intra professional cooperation and multidisciplinary partnership" (Lachman, 2015, p. 40).
- **Provision 3.5: Acting on Questionable Practice**—Outlines that nurses are obligated to "recognize and take action concerning any occurrences 'of incompetent, un-ethical, illegal or impaired practice by any member of the health care team . . .'" (Lachman, 2015, p. 40). This provision further states that nurses are expected to "express their concern to the persons observed with the questionable

practice and, if needed to resolve the situation, direct their concern to an administrator" (Lachman, 2015, p. 40). This specifies that incivility, bullying, and horizontal/lateral violence are unethical. This provision also mandates that the health care facility should also hold an ethical responsibility to address any practice that violates the code of conduct.

- **Provision 3.6: Addressing Impaired Practice**—The ANA does not view any nurse having a drug or alcohol problem or mental or physical illness just as a colleague who is impaired, but as a person whom the facility identifies as one who needs help in managing his or her life in a more effectual manner. "Incivility, bullying and horizontal/lateral violence affect the work climate, job performance, and satisfaction of all who are impacted by such behaviors" (Lachman, 2015, p. 40).

ZERO TOLERANCE MAY HAVE ZERO EFFECTIVENESS

Nursing and health care leaders including the ANA often leap immediately to declare that their facility follows a "zero-tolerance" policy when dealing with bullying or that only zero tolerance to bullying will eliminate it. The literature, however, reveals that this implementation rarely succeeds when used in isolation. One reason is that those enforcing the zero tolerance are bullies themselves.

Despite several studies that state that a "culture of zero tolerance for horizontal violence is the most effective leadership strategy to prevent its occurrence" (Longo & Sherman, 2007, p. 50), there are initial steps that must be taken before a zero-tolerance policy is introduced to the staff and enforced, especially among staff members who have tolerated bullying for some time. These are discussed in Chapter 8.

A FIELD GUIDE TO BULLYING AND INCIVILITY

This text is intended to act as a field guide to bullying and incivility in nursing. It will help you to recognize when it occurs, assist those who are victims, and develop policies and procedures to eliminate bullying and incivility from your workplace. This text outlines the provisions brought forth in the ANA position statement on bullying, incivility, and workplace violence, including definitions, recommendations, responsibilities, and resources.

References

American Association of Colleges of Nursing. (2008). *The Essentials of Baccalaureate Education for Professional Nursing Practice*. Washington, DC: Author.

American Nurses Association. (2015a). *Incivility, bullying, and workplace violence*. Washington, DC: Author. Retrieved from http://www.nursingworld.org/MainMenuCategories/WorkplaceSafety/Healthy-Nurse/bullyingworkplaceviolence/Incivility-Bullying-and-Workplace-Violence.html

American Nurses Association. (2015b). *Code of ethics for nurses with interpretive statements*. Washington, DC: Author.

Ariza-Montez, A., Muniz, N. M., Montero-Simó, M. J., & Araque-Padilla, R. A. (2013). Workplace bullying among healthcare workers. *International Journal of Environmental Research and Public Health, 10*(8), 3121–3139. doi:10.3390/ijerph10083121

Castronovo, M. A., Pullizzi, A., & Evans, S. (2016). Nurse bullying: A review and a proposed solution. *Nursing Outlook, 64*, 208–214.

Dellasega, C. A. (2009). Bullying among nurses. *American Journal of Nursing, 109*(1), 52–58.

Gaffney, D. A., DeMarco, R. F., Hofmeyer, A., Vessey, J. A., & Budin, W. C. (2012). Making things right: Nurses' experience with workplace bullying—A grounded theory. *Nursing Research and Practice, 1*, 1–10.

Heathfield, S. M. (2016). How to deal with a bully at work: Don't be an easy target for a bully. Retrieved from http://www.thebalance.com

Lachman, V. D. (2015). Ethical issues in the disruptive behaviors of incivility, bullying, and horizontal/lateral violence. *Urology Nurse, 35*(1), 39–42.

Larson, J. (2013). Nursezone: Nurse bullying an ongoing problem in the health care workplace. Retrieved from http://www.workplacebullying.org

Longo, J., & Sherman, R. O. (2007). Leveling horizontal violence. *Nursing Management, 38*(3), 34–37, 50–51.

2

What Is a Bully?

The simple definition of a bully is anyone who uses his or her perceived strength or power to intimidate another person who, he or she thinks, is weaker in order to gain power over that person. However, the answer to the question What is a bully? varies among individuals based on their personal experiences, and a clear definition, among all those studying the behavior, cannot be agreed upon.

After reading this chapter, the reader will be able to:

- List the root causes of bullying
- Explain the way in which a child is raised can create an adult bully
- Explain how societal norms or what are commonly accepted by our culture fuel the bullying behavior
- Explain how girls/women are more often bullies than boys/men
- List categories of bullying
- List types of bullies

WHAT ARE THE ROOT CAUSES OF BULLYING?

Why do people become bullies? A person does not suddenly "become" a bully. There aren't "born" bullies—they become that way. Bullying is a learned behavior that without correction becomes, to the bullied, acceptable behavior. But how does this occur? What causes a person to bully?

If a person was bullied or verbally abused by his or her parents, he or she learns that this is an acceptable behavior. Beyond the home, our culture also influences behavior in individuals. Power and violence are often glorified and may be valued in a family or social group over weakness. Adult bullies begin as childhood bullies. Much attention has been paid to childhood bullies, but very little to adult ones.

BULLYING BROKEN DOWN

In order for the label of "bullying" or "bully" to be applied to a set of behaviors or to an individual, the frequency and length of time over which the action has occurred must be reviewed. For example, true bullying occurs regularly and repeatedly over a period of time. Following are the actions considered to be bullying:

- It can be physical or verbal
- It can include threats, exclusion, or violence
- It can take place in a single occurrence or over a period of time, by the same person or by a group
- It occurs throughout all age ranges and in all places: school, the workplace, social settings
- It can include recurrent efforts to inflict physical injury or emotional harm
- It can occur between strangers, work peers, acquaintances, or friends
- It is intentional
- It focuses on a specific target or targets
- It includes psychological cruelty and well-thought-out actions
- It is disruptive and interferes with work

Fast Facts in a Nutshell

Many bullies find support from those around them, thus validating the behavior. Those who approve the behavior provide a willing audience that further fuels the aggression. Often, those who do not want to be bullied become part of the group supporting the bully.

Children are especially vulnerable to the effects of bullying. If children:

- Witness a loved one being overpowered at home by abuse, they will attempt to exert power over others
- Feel a lack of attention or love at home, they may become angry and act out anger on others
- Are given every material possession or exist without rules or guidance from parents, they may feel that they have power over others because they have power over their parents to get what they want
- Endure a parenting style that is overly punitive, it thereby creates anger that they may take out on others
- Are socially rejected by other children and not included in activities, they may interact with other children in the same way by excluding others
- Are not strong academically, they are more prone to becoming bullies
- Had an attentive, loving home but were never taught empathy toward others, they will treat others without empathy

THE CHILDHOOD BULLY BECOMES AN ADULT BULLY

If the behavior of bullying is not corrected in a child, he or she grows up to bully others as adults. Societal norms or what are commonly accepted by our culture also fuel the bullying behavior. These "normal" behaviors include:

- The glorification of power and violence over those who are weak
- A place of employment that does not value how its employees are treated
- Negative behavior that gets more recognition than positive behavior
- Jealousy and envy of the successes or possessions of others
- Lack of empathy and social skills
- Employees placed in leadership positions without being properly educated in leadership skills
- Feeling of a real or sensed imbalance of power or conflict

IT IS A GIRL THING

"Men and boys express aggression more often through physical violence and girls and women express it through character defamation, humiliation, betrayal of trust, and exclusion" (Dellasega, 2009, p. 53). The reason why men and women express aggression differently has not been widely studied, although there are various hypotheses, such as:

- Evolutionary development—in ancient societies, males had to act aggressively to protect their families and villages. Women had to survive in order to protect and care for children, so women became the nonovertly aggressive of the sexes.
- Society and culture indirectly encourage acts of aggression in boys (playing with toy guns, contact sports, etc.) and discourage it in girls (playing more quiet games).
- Women are biologically/hormonally designed to respond to stress differently.
- Females, controlled by oxytocin and hormones, tend to respond to others with caregiving and attachment behaviors.

- Female aggression is not fueled by testosterone, which fuels male aggression.
- Female aggression is thought to be more "cerebral" than physical (Dellasega, 2009, p. 53).

SIGNS OF BULLYING

Just one incident of bullying does not indicate that the perpetrator is a bully or that the victim is being bullied. However, it can impact a nurse and the care he or she provides to patients. Bullying is intentional and ongoing; it is not done by "accident." It tends to progress over time and become more serious. According to Esther Chipps (Chipps & McRury, 2012), a clinical nurse scientist, bullying has four distinct features:

- **Intensity**—the number of acts of bullying committed
- **Repetition**—not an isolated act or a one-time interaction between the victim and the perpetrator
- **Duration**—the bullying occurs over a specific period of time
- **Power disparity**—the victim is unable to stop the abuse

CATEGORIES OF BULLYING

According to researchers, there are five categories of bullying outlined by Hinchberger (2009, p. 38):

- Threats to professional status (humiliation, belittling, saying someone "is lazy")
- Threats to personal standing (insults, name-calling, intimidation)
- Isolation (social, withholding information, prevention of access to opportunities)
- Overwork or undue pressure (prevention of completion of care, increased stress)
- Destabilization (failure to give credit where credit is due, setting someone up to fail)

TYPES OF BULLYING

Several terms are used to describe bullying and incivility in all professions including nursing. These terms, defined particularly for nursing, are:

- **Academic incivility**—behavior by student nurses in the classroom that interferes with teaching and learning
- **Physician disruptive behavior versus nurse disruptive behavior**—overt and direct versus passive-aggressive
- **Workplace mobbing**—used to describe a type of adult bullying in nursing
  - Includes behavior "that continuously and systematically intimidates, shows hostility, threatens, offends, humiliates, or insults a coworker; interferes with a coworker's performance; or has an adverse impact on a coworker's mental or physical well-being" (Hutton & Gates, 2008, p. 169)
  - Victim usually an outstanding worker
  - Seen predominantly in nursing academic settings and is caused by the "envy of excellence and jealousy associated with the achievements of others . . . it occurs in an attempt to maintain group mediocrity and compliance with the established status quo . . ." (ANA, 2015, p. 2)
  - Employed to keep the employee or employees "in line" and to keep the individual or group from succeeding or overachieving

Fast Facts in a Nutshell

Workplace mobbing "is used by a group of nurses who 'gang up' on a particular employee and subject them to 'psychological harassment that may result in severe psychological and occupational consequences for the victim'" (ANA, 2015, p. 2).

- **Relational aggression**—uses psychological and social behaviors rather than violence or overt aggression to cause psychological harm
  - Another type of bullying thought to be common in nursing
  - Occurs mainly among women
  - Takes place across all levels of a work hierarchy (unlike horizontal or lateral violence)
  - Also known as "covert" or "indirect" bullying, but these are misnomers as openly speaking in a degrading way about another coworker is hardly "covert"
  - Type of bullying occuring when staff nurses bully a new graduate or student nurse
  - May extend beyond the workplace
  - Occurs in social media
- **Workplace bullying**—means to encompass the entire work setting and all health care providers within the location
- **Workplace mistreatment**—term coined and used by authors Read and Laschinger in 2013 in their work "Correlates of new graduate nurses' experiences of workplace mistreatment" to note incivility and bullying in the workplace (as cited in Wright & Naresh, 2015, p. 140)
- **Vertical violence**—between nurses of unequal power levels, such as between a unit manager and a staff nurse or between a nursing instructor and a student
- **Horizontal violence or horizontal hostility**—between those of the same level of employment, such as between a staff nurse and a staff nurse or between an educator and an educator
  - Also known as "horizontal hostility," the behavior can be hidden and used to "control, diminish, or devalue an individual or group" (Hinchberger, 2009, p. 38)
  - Occurs within the same group or intergroup of nurses
  - Described as a symptom of the oppression and sense of powerlessness felt within a group (Hinchberger, 2009, p. 38)
  - ". . . depends on the relationships between the bullies with informal organizational alliances. These

relationships enable bullies to control work teams and to use emotional abuse and psychological violence (including destruction of self-confidence and self-image) to enforce their work rules" (Hinchberger, 2009, p. 41)

THE NEGATIVE EFFECTS OF BULLYING

Identified by Heinz Leymann (1996), bullying has five different effects on the victim. He or she struggles with:

- Communication
- The ability to maintain social contacts
- The ability to maintain personal reputation
- His or her poor occupational situation
- His or her physical health concerns

References

American Nurses Association. (2015). *Incivility, bullying, and workplace violence.* Washington, DC: Author. Retrieved from http://www.nursingworld.org/MainMenuCategories/WorkplaceSafety/Healthy-Nurse/bullyingworkplaceviolence/Incivility-Bullying-and-Workplace-Violence.html

Chipps, E. M., & McRury, M. (2012). The development of an educational intervention to address workplace bullying. *Journal for Nurses in Staff Development, 28*(3), 94–98.

Dellasega, C. A. (2009). Bullying among nurses. *American Journal of Nursing, 109*(1), 52–58. doi:10.1097/01.NAJ.0000344039.11651.08

Hinchberger, P. A. (2009). Violence against female student nurses in the workplace. *Nursing Forum, 44*(1), 38–46.

Hutton, S., & Gates, D. (2008). Workplace incivility and productivity losses among direct care staff. *Workplace Health & Safety, 56*(4), 168–175.

Leymann, H. (1996). *Mobbing and victimization at work*. Hove, UK: Psychology Press.

Wright, W., & Naresh, K. (2015). Bullying among nursing staff: Relationship with psychological/behavioral responses of nurses and medical errors. *Health Care Management Review, 40*(2), 139–147.

3

Incivility in Nursing

Latoya N. Rawlins

Nursing is a profession that is rooted in caring behaviors. We learn early in our nursing education that the hallmark of this profession is providing compassionate care, yet incidents of uncivil acts continue to surge in both academic and practice settings. These uncivil acts have detrimental effects on the nursing profession.

After reading this chapter, the reader will be able to:

- Define incivility in nursing
- Identify the relationship between incivility and stress
- List 10 examples of uncivil behaviors
- List five effects of incivility on the nursing profession
- Identify individual and organizational strategies to mitigate incivility

DEFINITION OF INCIVILITY IN NURSING

"Incivility" can be defined as rude, impolite, or disrespectful behaviors to others that may result in physical or physiological harm (Clark, 2009). These discourteous and ill-mannered behaviors may range from demeaning remarks to verbal threats to safety. The behaviors may be intentional or unintentional and have the ability to cause long-standing effects on victims.

Incivility in the practice setting may occur on a hierarchal or lateral level. Common occurrences of uncivil behaviors from supervisors/nurse managers to staff nurses, physicians to nurses, nurses to nurses, senior nurses to newly graduated nurses, and nurses to nursing students have been reported in the practice setting. In the academic setting, there are four main types of incivility: faculty-to-faculty, faculty-to-student, student-to-faculty, and student-to-student. Regardless of the setting or type of incivility, these behaviors are unacceptable in a profession that is dedicated to the care and well-being of others.

INCIVILITY AND STRESS

There is no excuse for incivility, but it is crucial to recognize that stressful environments breed uncivil behavior. In the practice setting, nurses are challenged with staffing shortages, high patient-to-nurse ratios, and physical and psychological demands of the profession.

In the academic settings, educators are strained by faculty shortages, unrealistic teaching workloads, stress from tenure and promotion requirements as well as from balancing teaching and scholarship and service obligations. Students have reported stress from heavy workload demands, a competitive educational environment, and financial difficulties. The personal demands of life must also be considered. People are more likely to act uncivil in stressful situations. Stress can cause loss of sleep, tension, distress, anxiety, irritability, and anger. This can lead to irrational behavior that may be displayed in the form of incivility. Academic and practice settings should recognize the relationship between high stress and the increased incidents of uncivil acts. Strategies to decrease stress and promote the health and wellness of employees and students should be incorporated in incivility elimination strategies.

Fast Facts in a Nutshell

Stress is a core catalyst of incivility in both academic-based and practice-based environments.

HOW IS INCIVILITY DIFFERENT FROM BULLYING?

Unlike incivility, bullying is considered a form of violence. It is:

- Purposeful
- Deliberate
- Intended to harm the receiver, either physically or psychologically

The perpetrator seeks to control the victim through hostile or intimidating acts. Incivility is often displayed as rude or disrespectful behavior from one person to another. Lack of respect, ineffective communication, and poor interpersonal relationships are often seen in uncivil acts. Moreover, incivility may be purposeful or accidental, whereas bullying is almost always premeditated and calculated.

Although incivility is often seen as rude, harmless behavior or a mild form of bullying, research has highlighted that uncivil behaviors may be intended and can be harmful to the recipient (Clark, 2008; Lashley & de Meneses, 2001). People who are uncivil display a lack of regard for others through direct and indirect behaviors. These seemingly subtle behaviors can be detrimental to the well-being of others. A main cause of concern is that uncivil acts that are not mitigated can escalate into bullying. What may have begun as gossiping or spreading rumors may eventually spiral into hostile or violent bullying behaviors if not resolved. It is pivotal that we create a zero-tolerance environment for both incivility and bullying in all realms of the nursing profession.

WHAT BEHAVIORS DEFINE INCIVILITY?

Incivility can be described in the following ways. It is:

- Covert
- Direct and blatant aggression
- Overt—more subtle behaviors such as sarcasm, gossiping, or gesturing
- From one person to another or between a group and a targeted person ("mobbing"); this is when a specific person is the victim of rude and discourteous behavior from two or more persons

Have you ever wondered if you work in an uncivil environment or if you have been unknowingly uncivil to others? Ask yourself these questions:

- Do I feel disrespected by anyone or have I disrespected anyone at work?
- Do I partake in or witness the spreading of rumors or gossip about others?
- Have I heard or made demeaning remarks about colleagues?
- Is technology used for reasons other than what is intended?
- Is lateness and absenteeism an issue in my workplace?
- Have I witnessed colleagues shouting at each other or demonstrating other forms of unprofessional communication?
- Have I witnessed or displayed disruptive or intimidating behaviors in the work environment?
- Am I a part of a clique or is my work environment divided into cliques?

The purpose of these questions is for self-reflection. Answering yes to any of the questions may indicate that you are indeed working in an uncivil environment or that you may have been intentionally or unintentionally committing uncivil acts. It is important to bring about awareness as uncivil behaviors are often inadvertent. Therefore, behaviors that are considered uncivil should be clearly delineated in both academic-based and practice-based settings. Uncivil behaviors may be manifested in many forms. Some behaviors that constitute incivility are:

- Withholding information that is necessary for patient care
- Making disrespectful or sarcastic remarks
- Being habitually late or absent
- Using cell phone/technology inappropriately
- Spreading rumors
- Threatening safety
- Intimidating behaviors
- Exercising poor e-mail etiquette
- Arguing/yelling or using foul language
- Making condescending or belittling remarks
- Displaying favoritism
- Manifesting gender bias or racial bias
- Making verbal insults
- Extending breaks or lunchtime with little regard for colleague or patient care/safety
- Discrediting others
- Texting or e-mailing during meetings
- Using social media during scheduled work time
- Using social media to post disrespectful or belittling comments about colleagues

The preceding list has examples of uncivil behaviors that may occur in both the practice and academic settings. The following list has examples of behaviors directly related to the academic setting:

- Discrediting an instructor
- Posting rude remarks in an online learning forum
- Cheating on examinations
- Subjective grading or evaluations
- Threatening to fail a student
- Sleeping in class
- Canceling class without prior notification
- Demanding faculty to change grades
- Using cell phone in class
- Having a sense of entitlement by students
- Having a sense of supremacy by faculty
- Engaging in side conversations during class
- Presenting ambiguous/unclear syllabus
- Acting in a way that disrupts the teaching–learning environment

HOW DOES INCIVILITY LEAD TO BULLYING?

Creating an environment that is free from harmful behaviors is the responsibility of everyone. Failure to address incivility when it occurs can lead to bullying behaviors. Small acts of rude behavior become bigger acts, which spiral along the incivility to bullying. Clark (2008) describes this as the "continuum of incivility" in which low-risk behaviors such as sarcastic remarks that are ignored propel into more high-risk behaviors such as physical violence. Perpetrators will only do things that they can get away with. Uncivil behaviors are intended to trigger a response or intimidate the recipient, and if the desired response is not received, the behaviors can progressively worsen. It is important to identify and address these behaviors in both the practice and academic settings before they escalate.

WHAT ARE THE EFFECTS OF INCIVILITY?

Incivility is known to have detrimental effects on one's physical and psychological health (Clark, 2008). Nurses have reported loss of sleep, depression, lack of motivation, and loss of wages due to uncivil acts, and some nurses have left the profession as a result of incivility (Lashley & de Meneses, 2001). Incivility not only affects victims but also has significant effects on the work environment by lowering morale and productivity.

In the academic setting, uncivil acts are disruptive to the teaching–learning environment. For example:

- Time is lost from teaching to address discourteous behaviors inside and outside of the classroom.
- Uncivil acts create distraction for other learners and have the potential to create a culture of disrespect in the classroom.
- Student nurses have reported lack of motivation, fear, anxiety, and transferring or leaving nursing programs as a result of faculty-to-student incivility.

In practice setting, incivility compromises patient safety. For example:

- Perpetrators of incivility tend to demonstrate aggressive behaviors, inefficient communication skills, and poor interprofessional collaboration.
- An uncivil work environment decreases the quality of care and increases the risk of medical errors and patient harm.
- Uncivil acts such as withholding information and failure to act can result in unfavorable outcomes for patients.
- Incivility is a financial burden for health care organizations because it has the potential to increase nurse turnover rates, litigations, and dissatisfaction for both patients and employees (Porath & Pearson, 2010).

These harmful effects have alarmed professional organizations to address the issue of incivility with a sense of urgency.

HOW TO INTERVENE?

As professional nurses, we have a responsibility to abide by the American Nurses Association (ANA) *Code of Ethics for Nurses with Interpretative Statements* and demonstrate behaviors that are kind and compassionate and free from harm for both patients and health care workers. Several provisions explain that nurses are obligated to demonstrate caring, compassionate, and respectful behaviors not just to patients but to all individuals as well (ANA, 2015a). These behaviors should be modeled in practice and academic settings. It is equally important to speak up when you witness or have been a victim of uncivil acts. Professional organizations are taking a stand against incivility in an effort to create safer practice and learning environments. ANA (2015b) developed the position statement titled *Incivility, Bullying, and Workplace Violence* as a call for action to address violence in nursing. The Joint Commission has called upon leaders of health care institutions to create a culture of safety that delivers quality care. It has established leadership standards that require health care organizations to create a code of conduct for employees with a clearly prescribed method to address disruptive and inappropriate behaviors (The Joint Commission, 2008). It is equally important to create a culture that allows the reporting of disruptive behavior without fear of retribution. The following can be done on an organizational level to create a sound culture for a health care organization:

- Establish a code of conduct for employee behaviors
- Behaviors that constitute incivility should be clearly outlined
- Create a reporting system that prevents retaliation
- Hold perpetrators accountable for uncivil acts
- Provide annual mandates for civility training

- Create a culture of zero tolerance for incivility; establish guidelines, policies, and procedures to support this environment

Classroom strategies to foster a civil environment:

- Establish expected behavioral and classroom norms
- Clearly delineate behaviors that are considered uncivil and repercussions in syllabus
- Be cognizant of sources of stress for both faculty and students
- Role-model civil behaviors in the classroom
- Create teaching–learning environment of mutual respect

Efforts as a group are crucial, but there is also an individual responsibility to protect patients as well as the practice and academic environment. Self-reflection and self-awareness are necessary to sustain a civil environment. Although acts of incivility can be purposeful, they are most often unintended. Maintaining awareness of one's behavior is the first step in creating change. Clark (2013) Workplace Civility Index is a tool that allows the examination of one's own behavior. It is a 20-item questionnaire designed for individuals to rate their behavior on a scale of 1 to 5. The maximum score is 100—the lower the score, the more uncivil the person. This tool is recommended as a starting point for self-assessment and self-awareness in an effort to identify uncivil behaviors and create change. Everyone should be held accountable to maintain a civil environment. The Clark Workplace Civility Index can be found at this website (www.ic4n.org/wp-content/uploads/2015/09/Clark-Workplace-Civility-Index-Revised-Likert.pdf).

Here are some simple things that you can do as an individual to create civil environments:

- Maintain self-awareness of your own behaviors
- Speak up when you witness uncivil behaviors

- Report inappropriate behaviors
- Adopt an attitude of zero tolerance for uncivil acts
- Be a role model for civility

Fast Facts in a Nutshell

We have an individual and social responsibility to maintain a culture of civility that provides quality care and does not compromise patient outcomes.

To act civilly is to behave in a manner that demonstrates courtesy and mutual respect for others. Recipients and observers of incivility often take a passive approach to handling uncivil behavior. This timid approach is not conducive to eliminating incivility. As nurses, we have a social responsibility to protect patients and demonstrate behaviors that are in accordance with the ANA *Code of Ethics for Nurses.* Incivility may lead to poor patient outcomes, moral distress, and ineffective team collaboration. Therefore, it is important to strive for civil academic and practice environments. Uncivil behaviors that are disregarded can escalate into bullying behaviors and/or serious acts of violence. The ultimate cost of incivility to the nursing profession is unsafe patient care and disastrous patient outcomes. Nurses need to work in cohesive environments that support interprofessional collaboration. Through teamwork, self-awareness, open communication, accountability, mutual respect, and the general desire to do good and not harm, a civil culture can flourish.

HOW TO PROMOTE CIVILITY

The ANA states that it is the responsibility of all nurses to model civil behavior. This can be done by using the following practices:

- Be sure that you are clear in your verbal communication
- Treat colleagues, patients, and their families with respect, dignity, and kindness
- Consider how your words affect others
- Avoid gossip and do not spread rumors
- Rely on facts, not rumors or conjecture
- Always collaborate and share important patient information
- Offer assistance to your colleagues; if offered assistance you do not require, refuse gracefully
- Take responsibility for your actions
- Know that abuse of power is never to be tolerated
- Always speak directly to the person who has hurt you or caused an issue
- Demonstrate a willingness to accept another person's point of view
- Be polite, respectful, and apologetic when necessary
- Encourage, support, and mentor other staff
- Actively listen to everyone with interest and respect
- Uphold the nursing code of ethics at all times

References

American Nurses Association. (2015a). *Code of ethics for nurses with interpretive statements*. Washington, DC: Author.

American Nurses Association. (2015b). *Incivility, bullying, and workplace violence*. Washington, DC: Author. Retrieved from http://www.nursingworld.org/MainMenuCategories/WorkplaceSafety/Healthy-Nurse/bullyingworkplaceviolence/Incivility-Bullying-and-Workplace-Violence.html

Clark, C. M. (2008). The dance of incivility in nursing education as described by nursing faculty and students. *Advances in Nursing Science*, *31*, 37–54.

Clark, C. M. (2009). Faculty field guide for promoting student civility. *Nurse Educator*, *34*(5), 194–197.

Clark, C. M. (2013). *Creating and sustaining civility in nursing education*. Indianapolis, IN: Sigma Theta Tau International.

The Joint Commission. (2008). *Behaviors that undermine a culture of safety.* Retrieved from http://www.jointcommission.org/assets/1/18/SEA_40.pdf

Lashley, F. R., & de Meneses, M. (2001). Student civility in nursing programs: A national survey. *Journal of Professional Nursing, 17,* 81–86.

Porath, C. L., & Pearson, C. M. (2010). The cost of bad behavior. *Organizational Dynamics, 39,* 64–71.

4

Bullying in Nursing

Why is it that, in a profession thought to be formed from individuals whose life goal is to care for others and show compassion, bullying is even discussed? When "bullying in nursing" is mentioned to those outside of the profession, it is usually met with a look of shock and verbalized disbelief. However, when it is discussed among fellow nurses, it is met with mutual agreement and a sharing of stories and an exclamation that it occurs not just on certain units, but among all nurses in all specialties of nursing and at all levels of the profession as well. But why do nurses bully? Surely, there has to be some deep-rooted reason. Does it originate prior to entering the profession or does it develop in nursing school or early in a nurse's career as a reaction to how he or she was treated? Is it a learned behavior? Many a nurse has wondered how the nurses with whom they work, who have dedicated their lives to caring for others, or educators, who have dedicated their lives to teach others to treat patients with kindness and concern, become bullies, often driving students, novice nurses, and experienced professionals out of the profession

After reading this chapter, the reader will be able to:

- List the actions of a nurse bully
- Explain two triggers of bullying in nursing
- Describe the patterns of bullying in nursing
- List 10 behaviors that indicate bullying in nursing
- Describe the nurse as "wounded healer"

DEFINITION OF A NURSE BULLY

A nurse bully is "a nurse who uses psychological and social harassment against another nurse through overt and covert behaviors" (Flateau-Lux & Gravel, 2014, p. 225). The American Nurses Association (ANA) defines bullying as "repeated, unwanted harmful actions intended to humiliate, offend, and cause distress in the recipient. Bullying actions include those that harm, undermine, and degrade" (ANA, 2015). "An unfortunate occurrence has been noted among those familiar with bullying in nursing . . . nurses often reject offers of assistance in dealing with the crisis," (Dellasega, 2009, p. 54).

Fast Facts in a Nutshell

"Bullying is allowed to occur for three reasons: because it can; because it is modeled; because it is left unchecked" (Clark & Ahten, 2011).

ACTIONS OF NURSE BULLY

The actions of a nurse bully include the following:

- Showing hostility
- Humiliating

- Getting up and leaving when the victim enters a room
- Acting out in anger and impatience
- If in management, directing the assignment of an unmanageable patient care load to the victim of his or her bullying
- If in management, assigning patient care that is either above or below the scope of practice of the victim
- If in management, not allowing another nurse to be promoted, take sick leave, take holiday time, or get overtime or compensation for work beyond a specific shift
- Delivering verbal attacks, taunts, insults; condescension in language and attitude
- Giving the silent treatment, such as excluding and ignoring
- Giving threats and intimidation
- Spreading rumors and lies that no one refutes
- Withholding support
- Giving work deadlines that are impossible to meet
- Withholding vital patient care information
- Ridiculing and humiliating the victim regarding his or her patient care
- Micromanaging
- Belittling and criticizing, faultfinding, and scapegoating
- Sabotaging the victim's work
- Refusing to help others in patient care
- If in management, removing or decreasing responsibilities from the victim
- Playing practical jokes that are excessive and hurtful
- Teasing and sarcasm
- If in management, being late or not showing up to meetings scheduled by others
- Coercing the victim to not take something to which he or she is entitled, such as a promotion or new position within the facility
- Ignoring policies and procedures
- Ignoring presentations given by others

- Demeaning those who pursue continuing education, and not appreciating experience
- Excluding others from social events outside the workplace

Fast Facts in a Nutshell

Bullying "... erodes your sense of comfort and security that you need to do your job in a professional manner" (Gaffney, DeMarco, Hofmeyer, Vessey, & Budin, 2012, p. 1).

VERBAL ABUSE

Another common type of bullying behavior in nursing is that of verbal abuse. One study conducted among pediatric nurses in 2005 revealed that 94% of them had experienced verbal abuse from coworkers, physicians, and patients (Chipps & McRury, 2012, p. 95). Another study conducted among Australian nurses broke down verbal abuse by the following types: rudeness (82%), shouting (68%), and sarcasm (64%; Chipps & McRury, 2012, p. 95). Verbal abuse can be "blatant or subtle and consists of communication through words, tone, or manner that disparages, intimidates, patronizes, threatens, accuses or disrespects another person" (Alspach, 2007, p. 12).

WHAT TRIGGERS BULLYING IN NURSING?

Bullying among nurses can be brought on by certain events or triggers (Dellasega, 2009, p. 54). These events or triggers include the following:

- Those who enter as new graduates, novice nurses, or student nurses (they are new, lack confidence, and feel powerless)

- Those who are perceived as being intelligent, competent, loyal, accomplished and who have integrity and who are dedicated to the unit/facility (Castronovo, Pullizzi, & Evans, 2016, p. 209)
- Those who think outside the box and have new ideas on how things should be; in other words, those who disturb the "status quo"
- Anyone whom someone at a higher level perceives as a threat to his or her comfortable status
- Being a seasoned nurse, but new to a unit or facility (he or she lacks confidence because of being new and not having friends or an advocate to assist him or her)
- Receiving a promotion or honor that another nurse feels is not deserved (Dellasega, 2009, p. 54)
- Having a previous issue in working well with others
- Receiving special attention from physicians (Dellasega, 2009, p. 54)
- Having to work on a unit that is severely short-staffed
- A lack of resources or equipment to properly and safely care for patients
- Working with violent or hostile patients and those with dementia
- Poor working relationship with colleagues
- Rapid changes within the facility or unit (i.e., change in governance, downsizing, restructuring)
- Low or nonexistent support from nursing leadership and facility administration
- Patient care "issues," such as excessive documentation, computer work, and shift "work" not completed and therefore passed on to the next shift
- Working the night shift, erroneously thought of as not working as hard as other shifts
- Aggressive behavior by another nurse triggering anger in a colleague: then anger triggers abrasive behavior in another colleague and the behavior is reinforced because it is ignored

PATTERNS OF BULLYING IN NURSING

Cheryl Dellasega in her article, "Bullying Among Nurses," notes that there are patterns to bullying in nursing. These are common to all specialties and all units. These types of behaviors tend to make other nurses on the unit feel intimidated or frustrated, even if they were not the ones being targeted for bullying (Dellasega, 2009, p. 54). See if you recognize yourself or nurses with whom you work in these patterns:

- **The Supernurse**
  - States she or he has seen and done it all in nursing and has performed better than coworkers and lords this over coworkers
  - Is usually more educated and experienced than his or her coworkers
  - Acts out feelings of superiority through verbal comments and body language (eye rolling, sighing)
  - Acts this way because he or she truly feels comments regarding the work of others are helpful
  - May be compensating for feelings of doubt, anxiety, and uncertainty
  - Is unaware of how his or her actions and verbalizations affect other nurses
- **The "PGR" Nurse**
  - Uses put downs, gossip, and rumors (PGR) to bully other nurses (Dellasega, 2009, p. 55)
  - Turns on other nurses instead of working with them through a stressful situation
  - Randomly selects and constantly changes those who are the target of their behavior
  - Responds aggressively and quickly to any remarks that he or she feels are hurtful, even when offense is not intended
  - May be trying to bond with other nurses through sharing of gossip and rumors—but the result of this behavior is still damaging to others

- **The Backstabbing Nurse**
    - Betrays the confidence and friendship of fellow nurses
    - Typically defined as "two faced"
    - Uses information about others to increase his or her "power" among fellow nurses; communication within the group can be misrepresented to others
    - Behaves in such a way that creates mistrust and affects working relationships
- **The Green With Envy Nurse**
    - Wants what he or she does not have either personally or professionally
    - Expresses his or her envy through comments or unhelpful behavior
    - Hides feelings of resentment from those he or she has targeted
- **The Clique Nurse**
    - Excludes other nurses as a form of antagonism
    - When two or more nurses form a group and exclude others—a clique can be a group of friends but it becomes harmful when they exclude others, show favoritism, help only those in the group, or ignore other nurses
    - Cliques are a "power base" and give the group a perceived "safe space"
    - The formation of a clique can be inadvertent, but it is a gathering of a subgroup of people

It should also be noted that bullies can develop because nurses of different ages have different approaches to patient care and can be intolerant of the new ideas or practices of the student, novice nurse, or newly employed nurse. Nurses who have been in the profession longer may also mimic the bullying behaviors that they experienced in the past. Nurse bullies, or any bully, can see the behavior in other nurses, but fail to see bullying behavior in themselves. They are among those who accept the behavior as normal. Bullies may also be seen by nursing leadership as those with "passion" and fail to confront the behavior.

SO, YOU THINK YOU ARE NOT A BULLY

Many of us know a bully but are convinced that we are not bullies ourselves. The checklist denotes the behavior of a nurse bully. Think about your behavior with your coworkers for a given time period. Have you demonstrated any of these behaviors?

- ☐ Withholding patient care information from a fellow nurse
- ☐ Gossiping and spreading rumors
- ☐ Sharing private information not meant to be shared
- ☐ Hiding patient care items from another nurse so that he or she is unable to care for the patient
- ☐ Establishing and maintaining cliques
- ☐ Ignoring another nurse who approaches a group that has gathered
- ☐ Ignoring the opinions of others
- ☐ Excluding another nurse from your social group
- ☐ Shouting at another nurse
- ☐ Publicly humiliating or ridiculing another nurse
- ☐ "Micromanaging" the work of another nurse or coworker
- ☐ Reminding another nurse of a past error
- ☐ Do fellow staff avoid you?
- ☐ Are your fellow staff angry or hurt by something you said?
- ☐ Do you praise fellow staff or just comment on their shortcomings or something they did wrong?
- ☐ Do you feel underqualified or over your head, and as a consequence place your staff in uncomfortable situations?

Checking off any of the these behaviors means that you act aggressively toward your fellow nurses and you are a bully.

THEORIES OF BULLYING IN NURSING

There are many posed theories regarding what causes a nurse to bully. Some postulate that it is a cycle, perpetually fueled by how nurses view themselves and other nurses. Others view bullying as a reaction to working conditions. These theories focus on how nurses view themselves, how they view other nurses, and how their training affects these views.

How Nurses View Themselves

The typical nurse is a young female who values "patient care, service and self-sacrifice" (Hurley, 2006, p. 69). Historically, nurses have been seen as being less mature and knowledgeable (read: "smart") regarding skill and reasoning ability and possessing less societal power than those who enter the field of medicine. Therefore, nurses are seen by society and unfortunately themselves as "lacking power, autonomy and self-esteem . . . they became marginalized and look to those whom they perceive as more powerful for approval" (Hurley, 2006, p. 69). "Nurses have existed for centuries within a system headed by male physicians, administrators, and marginalized female nurse managers" (Longo & Sherman, 2007, p. 35).

How Nurses View Other Nurses

Some nurses value other nurses who finish their tasks and assigned care "on time." The nurse who spends what others feel is "too long" interacting with a patient or completing care faces the consequences meted out by the peers. This can range from forcing the nurse to miss a meal due to increased workload to outright reprimand (Hurley, 2006, p. 69). But the person who is reprimanded feels that he or she cannot speak out against the perpetrator because the perpetrator is the "go to" person on the unit whom the nurse, particularly the new nurse, looks up to as a source of knowledge (Hurley, 2006, p. 69).

The Student Nurse

Student nurses "learn" to be submissive. A 2006 study noted that nursing students finish their degree programs with lowered self-esteem due to their treatment in nursing school. They then enter the field with their sense of autonomy affected and their competence level questioned by others and themselves. In order to survive, new nurses take on the submissive role to those who they feel have power over them (staff nurse, nurse managers, and physicians). Those who have the "power" often abuse those in submissive positions. It is also theorized that the student nurse, the oppressed, takes on the role of the oppressor in order to "survive." This internalized oppression also makes students, or new nurses, feel that there is no way to change the system in which they are now caught up. They now become the bullies they feared (Hurley, 2006).

Fast Facts in a Nutshell

Another typical target of a bully is a nurse who is experienced, highly educated, and clinically competent. It is unfortunate that bullying occurs across a nurse's career from being novice to expert.

THE PERPETUAL CYCLE OF BULLYING

So when viewed in its total context, bullying and the outcomes of the bullying behavior cause a cycle that must be broken. The nurse feels that he or she is being oppressed by the system, and by internalized feelings of low self-esteem (caused by being bullied, derided, and disrespected by physicians, instructors, managers, and fellow nurses). Nurses feel powerless to control their working conditions; they feel a lack of autonomy. Rather than asserting themselves and standing up to the system, fellow nurses, and managers and risking revenge by them, the oppressed nurses act out their feelings by bullying others, because that behavior is covert and free from penalty. The victims fear retribution and the possibility of losing their source of knowledge and help on the unit. They become distressed, helpless, and powerless, and thus the cycle continues.

THE NURSE AS WOUNDED HEALER

Nurses become nurses for many different reasons such as helping other people who are suffering. Many nurses are drawn to the profession after experiencing or witnessing a physically or verbally traumatic event in their own lives either personally or through their work (Christie & Jones, 2014). How the nurse coped with the previous traumatic experience determines how she or he will cope with all future experiences. The theory of the "Nurse as Wounded Healer" was developed by Conti-O'Hare in 2002. In it, she states that if a nurse forms healthy coping mechanisms to deal with the trauma, she is termed "the wounded healer."

- The trauma has been recognized and dealt with and the nurse has healed and uses past experience to assist him or her in dealing with future traumas and to assist others.
- The nurse is able to empathize with the patients and their colleagues.
- The nurse helps to create positive work environments.
- The nurse utilizes the self as a therapeutic tool to help others.

If the coping mechanisms were ineffective, the nurse is termed "the walking wounded."

- The trauma has not been recognized and dealt with and the nurse has not healed and does not use past experiences to assist him or her in dealing with future traumas and to assist others.

- The pain and trauma of a past experience goes on to affect the nurse's social and work relationships.
- The nurse feels anger and has emotional problems.
- The nurse's past psychological "wounds" are projected onto patients and colleagues and make him or her less able to be empathetic (Christie & Jones, 2014).
- The nurse often deals with alcohol and drug abuse.
- The nurse suffers from job dissatisfaction and burnout.
- The nurse exists in a negative work environment.

Nurses face so many stresses in their daily work and personal lives. The nurse who is among the "walking wounded" is unable to cope with these stressors without the use of a healthy outlet (which they have not learned to find). Colleagues, whom they perceive as weak and indefensible, become the targets of their misplaced aggression. If the victim does not have effective coping mechanisms, or fails to confront the bully, he or she becomes the "walking wounded" and the cycle continues.

References

Alspach, G. (Ed.). (2007). Are our interactions nice or nasty? *Critical Care Nurse, 27*(3), 10–14.

American Nurses Association. (2015). *Incivility, bullying, and workplace violence.* Washington, DC: Author. Retrieved from http://www.nursingworld.org/MainMenuCategories/WorkplaceSafety/Healthy-Nurse/bullyingworkplaceviolence/Incivility-Bullying-and-Workplace-Violence.html

Castronovo, M. A., Pullizzi, A., & Evans, S. (2016). Nurse bullying: A review and a proposed solution. *Nursing Outlook, 64*, 208–214.

Conti-O'Hare, M. (n.d.). The theory of the nurse as wounded healer: Finding the essence of therapeutic self. Retrieved from http://cc.bingj.com/cache.aspx?q=Conti-O%e2%80%99Hare%2c+M.+(n.d.).+The+theory+of+the+nurse+as+wounded+healer%3a&d=4550493777428586&mkt=en-US&setlang=en-US&w=kU1zLmXjr9wVUwTV6HgSUJRQku6FrZey

Chipps, E. M., & McRury, M. (2012). The development of an educational intervention to address workplace bullying. *Journal for Nurses in Staff Development, 28*(3), 94–98.

Christie, W., & Jones, S. (2014). Lateral violence in nursing and the theory of the nurse as wounded healer. *Online Journal of Issues in Nursing, 19,* 1–11. Retrieved from http://www.nursingworld.org

Clark, C., & Ahten, S. (2011, August 19). Nurses: Resetting the civility conversation. *Nursing Outlook, 59*(3), 158–165.

Dellasega, C. A. (2009). Bullying among nurses. *American Journal of Nursing, 109*(1), 52–58.

Flateau-Lux, L. R., & Gravel, G. (2014). Put a stop to bullying new nurses. *Home Healthcare Nurse 32*(4), 225–229.

Gaffney, D. A., DeMarco, R. F., Hofmeyer, A., Vessey, J. A., & Budin, W. C. (2012). Making things right: Nurses' experience with workplace bullying—A grounded theory. *Nursing Research and Practice, 1,* 1–10.

Hurley, J. E. (2006). Nurse-to-nurse horizontal violence: Recognizing it and preventing it. *National Student Nurses' Association Imprint, 53*(4), 68–71.

Longo, J., & Sherman, R. O. (2007, March). Leveling horizontal violence. *Nursing Management, 38*(3), 34–37, 50–51.

5

Understanding Workplace Violence in Health Care

Each year, the U.S. Bureau of Labor Statistics releases a report analyzing injuries and illnesses that result in time away from work. In 2013, 13% of days away from work in the health care and social assistance sector were the result of violence, and this rate has continued to increase. Violence has not escaped the nursing profession. In a recent survey of 3,765 registered nurses and nursing students, the American Nurses Association (ANA) noted that "43% of respondents have been verbally and/or physically threatened by a patient or family member of a patient. Additionally, 24% of respondents have been physically assaulted by a patient or family member of a patient while at work" (ANA, 2015, p. 4).

After reading this chapter, the reader will be able to:

- List the five "building blocks" of an Occupational Safety and Health Administration (OSHA) workplace violence prevention program
- Name three risks of workplace violence
- List engineering controls to prevent workplace violence

(*continued*)

- List five administrative controls to prevent workplace violence
- List five topics of safety education and training

WORKPLACE VIOLENCE DEFINED

Many professional organizations have sought to define workplace violence; however, the OSHA defines workplace violence as "violent acts, including physical assaults and threats of assault, directed towards persons at work or on duty" (OSHA, 2015a). This is an umbrella definition that includes physical assault or threats that can result in physical harm. Those who have developed prevention and treatment programs concerning workplace violence have broadened this to include verbal violence—"threats, verbal abuse, hostility, and harassment" (OSHA, 2015a). This then indicates that even if the behavior does not cause physical harm, it can cause psychological trauma and stress. It is known that verbal assault can escalate into physical violence.

Fast Facts in a Nutshell

"From 2002 to 2013 incidents of workplace violence . . . were four times more common in healthcare than in the private industry on average" (OSHA, 2015a).

SOURCES OF POTENTIAL VIOLENCE

In 2013, "80% of serious violent incidents reported in healthcare settings were caused by interactions with patients" (OSHA, 2015a). Other sources included outside customers, students, coworkers, and facility intruders. According to Hinchberger, the health care areas with highest incidents of violence include (2009, p. 40):

- Emergency department—12% of emergency room (ER) nurses experienced physical violence (Hinchberger, 2009)
- Waiting rooms
- Psychiatric wards
- Geriatric units

According to a U.S. Bureau of Labor Statistics report in 2013, the highest rate of violence against health care workers was against psychiatric aides, that is, there were 590 injuries per 10,000 full-time employees. This figure was 10 times higher than that of another group of victims, nursing assistants. There were 55 injuries per 10,000 full-time employees in this group. Those who experienced workplace violence were kicked, hit, beaten, and shoved. It is unfortunate to consider that the high number of workplace violence incidents includes only those where workers reported time away from work.

Fast Facts in a Nutshell

The largest source of violence to health care providers (ambulatory care centers, hospitals, long-term care, and residential care facilities) is patients.

A vast number of incidents go unreported even in facilities that have a formal reporting system. Incidents are underreported due to a lack of reporting policy, a lack of faith in the reporting system, and a fear of retaliation (OSHA, 2015a). Those in health care may be reluctant to report violence because they feel that violence is an expected part of their job. They may feel that it is a result of a patient's illness or condition that makes him or her violent; therefore, a workplace injury is expected. Nurses also do not wish to label patients as being impaired or that they are violent.

SUGGESTED SAFETY MEASURES TO DECREASE WORKPLACE VIOLENCE

The American Federation of State, County and Municipal Employees has outlined some ideas that would reduce health care facility violence (Hinchberger, 2009, p. 44). These include:

- Restrict access to facility buildings, especially during evening- and night-shift hours
- Install locks or security pass access on doors that lead to staff-only restricted areas
- Ensure that staff use ID badges that contain minimal identifying information
- Arrange security distribution of visitor passes
- Ensure that sharps and other tools that could be used to harm another person be kept locked
- Install panic alarms in areas where staff may interact with the public
- Allow use of mobile phones and pagers
- Provide adequate staffing
- Implement a "buddy system"
- Provide security escorts to parking areas especially during evening and night shift
- Provide training in defusing violent situations, self-defense, and unit/facility escape routes
- Ensure that nurses should be mindful of the importance of providing timely information to significant others or patients who are waiting, and staff should also be mindful of how a patient or significant other may react when receiving sensitive information
- Use common sense or "evidence-based practices" in reducing wait times in patient care areas or during patient care

OSHA GUIDELINES TO REDUCE VIOLENCE IN HEALTH CARE SETTINGS

In 1970, OSHA put forth a requirement for all employers, called the General Duty Clause. This clause states that all employers have a duty to "furnish to each of his employees a place of employment which is free from recognized hazards that are causing or are likely to cause death or a serious physical harm" (OSHA, 2015b). OSHA has developed a workplace violence prevention program that has five core "building blocks." These building blocks are:

- Management commitment and employee participation
- Worksite analysis and hazard identification
- Hazard prevention and control
- Safety and health training
- Recordkeeping and program evaluation

MANAGEMENT COMMITMENT AND EMPLOYEE PARTICIPATION

Some facilities become serious about developing an anti-workplace violence program when the unthinkable happens within the facility or something is seen on the news that hits too close to home.

Fast Facts in a Nutshell

The average cost of caring for a nurse injured by workplace violence is $94,160.

What is universally needed in all facilities is management that is committed to the success of the program. Managers must consistently voice that aggressive or violent behavior is unacceptable and will result in suitable penalties. They must also commit to an environment where it is safe for employees and others to report aggressive and violent behavior.

- Antiviolence policies must be posted prominently throughout health care facilities so that they are visible to all employees and visitors.
    - The policy must contain the clearly stated position of the facility on workplace violence as well as the consequences that will be suffered for a policy violation.
    - The expected conduct and responsibilities of all staff and visitors should also be posted.
- Appropriate action after an incident should be visible to all staff so that trust is formed between the staff and the management, allaying fears of retribution. This will ensure staff that if an incident is witnessed or reported, proper action will take place.
- All staff should be involved in the creation of the antiviolence policies. Direct bedside staff is especially important for this group. Other members should include human resources, security, safety, legal departments, and unions, if applicable.
- Outside assistance in policy and procedure formation can be obtained from local law enforcement personnel.

WORKSITE ANALYSIS AND HAZARD IDENTIFICATION

It is important that management be continually aware of new hazards within facilities. All levels of management should collaboratively work with both direct patient care staff and nonclinical employees to assess safety risks. Assessment should include record review (violence-related records, OSHA forms, injury reports, incident reports, police reports, daily and event logs), patient record review, review of current policies and procedures for different job descriptions, results of employee and patient surveys (useful in monitoring whether the previous implemented safety measures are being followed or whether there are issues with their implementation), and ongoing security analysis.

Unscheduled and scheduled walk-throughs of a facility (including outside areas such as parking lots, parking garages, loading docks, and exterior buildings) are also useful to identify safety hazards. The walk-through should include staff who are a part of the workplace violence committee. Comprehensive follow-up of assessment findings should be completed and reported to appropriate personnel. OSHA has noted that there are several risk factors that could lead to violence in the workplace:

- Working with patients who have a history of violence, including those who suffer from substance abuse, gang members, and distraught patient family members and friends
- Working alone within a specific area of a health care facility or within the patient home
- Design of a health care unit that blocks the vision of the employee, not allowing direct supervision or not being conducive to staff escape from violence
- Poorly lit parking lots, hallways, nonpatient care rooms, and other areas
- No means for emergency communication among staff
- The presence of concealed weapons among patients and their visitors
- A facility in a high-crime area

There are several risk factors that management may be unaware of but that need to be addressed at a leadership level:

- Lack of policies and procedures for "recognizing and managing escalating hostile and assaultive behaviors from patients, clients, visitors or staff" (OSHA, 2015a)
- Lack of staff education in "recognizing and managing escalating hostile and assaultive behaviors from patients, clients, visitors or staff" (OSHA, 2015a)

- Allowing staff to work short-staffed—especially during high-risk times such as meal service, visiting hours, and night shift
- Inadequate security
- Inadequate mental health personnel
- Overcrowded, uncomfortable waiting areas with long waits for care
- The public being allowed to move unrestricted in a facility including patient care areas
- Public and staff having the perception that violence is tolerated and would not be reported
- "An overemphasis on customer satisfaction over staff safety" (OSHA, 2015a)

HAZARD PREVENTION AND CONTROL

This is the third step in the process of assessing a facility for issues concerning workplace violence. It should take place after a record review and facility walk-through. Once facility management is aware of the potential hazards, it can work to implement plans to correct the situation. The first step to mitigate a potential workplace violence hazard is to eliminate it altogether. For example, if a facility does not employ the appropriate staff specialty and/or numbers to safely care for psychiatric patients, then the facility should not admit them. Hazard prevention and control have two categories: engineering controls and administrative and work practice controls. These controls are best used in combination to more effectively prevent and control workplace violence.

Engineering controls include:

- Making exits more accessible by changing unit floor plans
- Removing physical barriers that block view of patients and visitors from staff
- Improving lighting in remote or outdoor areas

- Installing mirrors that allow staff to see around corridor corners
- Updating security hardware to include metal detectors, surveillance cameras, and panic buttons
- Controlling who is allowed to enter patient care areas, such as the ICU, ER, maternity units, and pediatric units
- Fully enclosing the nurses station or installing wide counters
- Replacing freely movable furniture (i.e., rolling office chairs) with immovable furniture—to prevent the furniture from being used as a weapon

Administrative and work practice controls include changing how staff members complete their assignments in order to prevent a violent incident and also what to do in case an incident should occur. This step is important when engineering controls are not possible or will not completely protect staff. Be mindful that what may work for one facility in a particular setting may not work for another in another setting. Implementation of controls should be balanced with "maintaining a calming, welcoming, and workable environment for staff, patients, and visitors" (OSHA, 2015a). Once implemented, however, the work is not done. Assessment and reassessment should be ongoing to ensure that the measures are satisfactory and that there are not any new threats requiring a change in policy or controls. Administrative controls include the following:

- Assessing and reassessing patients for potential violent behavior
    - Can be done on admission and periodically throughout the patient's stay
    - Include job status, financial situation, and psychological, social, and physical assessments
    - Should also include history of drug and alcohol abuse, history of violence, and arrest record

- Development of a procedure to track and communicate patient behavioral information among appropriate staff
- Develop special procedures for patients determined to be at high risk for violence
- Maintain adequate staffing for all units and shifts
- Provide training for all staff in "de-escalation techniques, workplace safety practices, and trauma-informed care" (OSHA, 2015a)—the long-term effect of physical, psychosocial, and emotional trauma on a survivor and how to avoid retraumatization
- Emergency procedures for all staff
- How to minimize stress on patients and visitors
- If a violence incident occurs ensure that medical and/or mental health care services and employee assistance programs are provided and that a postincident debriefing takes place where root cause analysis begins "that considers what happened, what should have happened, why the difference, and how to prevent a similar problem in the future" (OSHA, 2015b)

SAFETY AND HEALTH TRAINING

In order for any workplace violence prevention program to be successful, education and training of all staff are essential. Training should be specific to the unit and type of care the patients receive. All staff needs to be able to recognize a potential hazard and to protect themselves should a situation occur. Education should also emphasize that "violence is not an acceptable part of healthcare work" (OSHA, 2015b). Education and training should take place at orientation as needed or "just in time" or as part of web-based programs and then yearly or as appropriate. Topics should include the following:

- A general review of the facility/unit workplace violence prevention policies and procedures
- How and when to obtain a patient's risk profile

- Risk factors that can contribute to violence
- Policies and procedures for the assessment and documentation of a patient's change in behavior
- "Location, operation and coverage of safety devices such as alarm systems, along with the required maintenance schedules and procedures" (OSHA, 2015a)
- How to recognize when patient or visitor behavior escalates—warning signs or situations that lead to violent behavior
- How to prevent or diffuse volatile situations or aggressive behavior in patients, staff, visitors, and intruders
- The location and how to use safe rooms or areas of refuge
- The review of a standard response (i.e., code), including how to implement and who should respond and how
- Responsibility of all staff—directly and indirectly involved—regarding a workplace violence incident
- Self-defense methods and how to protect visitors, staff, and visitors
- Use of physical and chemical restraints—proper use, safety, and when to use
- How to report an incident and how to document it
- Procedure for obtaining medical care, counseling, workers' compensation, or legal assistance after an incident of workplace violence
- If using a prepackaged education/training program, include unit/facility-specific information
- All programs should include the following: patient versus employee, employee versus employee, and employee versus patient. Also review domestic violence and theft
- Opportunities to role-play and practice skills and competency measurement

RECORDKEEPING AND PROGRAM EVALUATION

An element that is essential in the evaluation of a workplace violence prevention program is recordkeeping and evaluation.

They assist in identifying hazards, determining additional measures that should be implemented, and keeping the program current and updated. Changes and updates to an existing program should be freely communicated to all levels of staff. Staff should be encouraged to suggest changes or updates based on their experiences and observations. Regular meetings of the workplace violence committee and its subgroups should take place.

Reporting of incidents (assaults, safety hazards, patient histories, staff education and training, and corrective actions after an incident) should include the following:

- The severity of a workplace violence incident or problem
- Identification of any trends or patterns on a particular unit, within a patient group, facility location, job classification, or specific department
- Methods used to evaluate hazard control
- Assessment of workplace violence prevention programs
- Identification of education and training needs

According to OSHA Regulation 29 CFR 1904, health care establishments are required to record and report work-related injury and illness (some medical offices or those facilities with 10 or fewer employees are exempt). This includes injury and illness that are "caused, contributed to, or significantly aggravated by events or exposures in the work environment." Incidents that must be reported include the following:

- Death
- Lost work days
- Restricted work
- Job transfer
- Medical treatment beyond basic first aid
- Loss of consciousness
- Significant injury or illness (e.g., cancer, broken bones, chronic disease)

Workplace violence program evaluation should include the following:

- Definition of violence, reporting system, and schedule of report review
- Staff meeting minutes or other reports that contain a review of ongoing safety and security issues
- Analyzing reports and incidents for trends in relation to baseline levels and the reporting of the same
- Measuring and reporting improvement or increase in incidents
- Maintaining records regarding administrative and workplace changes and the evaluation of programs
- Surveys of patients, visitors, and staff and their results
- Recommendations and their follow-through
- Seeking updated strategies to prevent violence
- OSHA and state regulatory compliance for illness/injury reporting
- Relationship with local law enforcement to foster ongoing education regarding workplace violence
- Requesting of consultation to review the facility for improvement

Records that should be reviewed include the following:

- All OSHA and state-required reports
- Workers' compensation reports
- Incident reports
- Reports of assault
- Abuse and aggressive behavior or other forms of violence
- Charts of patients who have a history of violence, drug and alcohol abuse, or who have been involved in criminal activities
- Minutes of safety meetings
- Records of training and education meetings, who attended the meetings, and qualifications of the trainers who provided training at the meetings

References

American Nurses Association. (2015). *Incivility, bullying, and workplace violence*. Washington, DC: Author. Retrieved from http://www.nursingworld.org/MainMenuCategories/WorkplaceSafety/Healthy-Nurse/bullyingworkplaceviolence/Incivility-Bullying-and-Workplace-Violence.html

Hinchberger, P. A. (2009). Violence against female student nurses in the workplace. *Nursing Forum*, *44*(1), 38–46.

Occupational Safety and Health Administration. (2015a). *Workplace violence in healthcare* (OSHA 3826). Retrieved from https://www.osha.gov

Occupational Safety and Health Administration. (2015b). *Preventing workplace violence: A road map for healthcare facilities* (OSHA 3827). Retrieved from https://www.osha.gov

6

The Cost of Nurse Bullying on the Health Care System

In a 2005 survey, 94% of nurses responded that the disruptive behavior of bullying had a negative effect on patient outcomes (Chipps & McRury, 2012, p. 95). This included adverse patient events, medication and treatment errors, altered patient safety, decreased quality of patient care, patient mortality, and decreased patient satisfaction (Chipps & McRury, 2012, p. 95). The effects of nurses being bullied spill over into the general health care system—first by unit, then by facility—affecting both patients and their significant others and ultimately hurting nursing's reputation among the general public. In other words, what affects the individual nurse affects the entire health care system and the quality of care patients receive.

After reading this chapter, the reader will be able to:

- List the ways bullying affects the health care system
- Describe how bullying affects the health care system
- Describe three ways bullying affects the health care system financially

(*continued*)

- Describe how bullying in nursing affects recruiting nurses
- Describe how bullying in nursing leads to medication errors

HOW DOES BULLYING AFFECT THE HEALTH CARE SYSTEM?

Nurses are the mainstay of the health care system. Anything that affects their ability to perform optimum patient care will affect the unit, facility, and overall health care of the nation. Bullying, incivility, and workplace violence are three issues that affect patient care. However, forms of bullying are not discussed very often because they may reveal an aspect of nursing that the health care system does not want exposed. The following are examples of how patient care is directly affected by bullying:

- Increased absenteeism occurs because of staff taking "mental health days" or due to illness or depression. Absenteeism leads to overall staffing shortages affecting patient care and increasing the stress on the remaining members of the staff, thus increasing bullying
- Decreased staff retention occurs as the bullied nurses come and go practically through a revolving door. The problem of the individual bully or bullies is never addressed; staffing shortages ensue, leading to stress on the remaining staff and to altered patient care.
- Staff nurses do not report issues or problems that affect their care of patients
- Decreased productivity occurs both in terms of the victim and those perpetrating the act as time is spent on dealing with the bullying behavior rather than caring for patients or educating nurses
- Disruption of professional relationships and cooperation leads to decreased communication and poor patient care

- Decreased cooperation among health care staff leads to decreased effectiveness of team work and dangerous conditions for the care of the patient
- Those who are bullied do not ask for help or guidance in a new patient care situation, leading to errors and patient harm. This includes moving debilitated patients on their own and using unfamiliar medical equipment.
- Management is distracted from dealing with issues of bullying and incivility (managing the situation, interviewing staff/witnesses, and then dealing with the results of lost employees: recruiting, interviewing, hiring, and training new staff)
- Ethical standards are lowered
- Medication errors increase because those intimidated by either a nurse's or a physician's past bullying behavior are reluctant to clarify orders (Chipps & McRury, 2012, p. 95). Medication errors also occur because the victim is mentally distracted due to bullying or the intimidating behavior of other nurses and physicians.
- A poor work environment due to bullying increases the chances of patient death and failure to rescue (Castronovo, Pullizzi, & Evans, 2016, p. 210)

OTHER ISSUES THAT AFFECT A HEALTH CARE INSTITUTION

- Student nurses on their clinical rotations see how staff treat each other and their fellow students; a unit where bullying is tolerated is not viewed as a viable future employer
- Decreased "customer service" and decreased enthusiasm regarding employment at a facility or on a particular unit among current nurses leads to decreased recruitment
- Morale is lowered
- Commitment to the health care organization or institution is decreased
- Attrition/resignation occurs

- New staff feel powerless to "fix" the corrupt system, being told "that's how it's always been done." They leave the unit/facility without explanation or an honest discussion of how bullying affected their decision.
- There can be incidents of suicide

Fast Facts in a Nutshell

Nurses agree that if you want respect in your job, do not become a nurse.

BY THE NUMBERS

Incivility and bullying affect not only the individual nurse and the immediate health care team, but also the facility in which they are employed, the patients cared for within, and the reputation of nursing as a whole. There is a correlation between decreased job productivity and dealing with incivility and bullying and patient care outcomes. For example, nursing assistants who were bullied did not complete assigned tasks, such as turning patients, providing hygiene, and assisting with ambulation. When these basic services are not provided in patient care, they can result in negative patient outcomes that prolong hospital stays (Hutton & Gates, 2008, p. 174). Many hospitals and health care systems act only on a problematic issue when it affects their bottom line. Bullying affects that as well.

- Seventy-eight percent of nurses report a decrease in their commitment to their work (Hunt & Zopito, 2012, p. 367)
- Eighty percent report a decrease in productivity because they are worried about an incident involving incivility or bullying (Hunt & Zopito, 2012, p. 367)
- Forty-five percent of U.S. workers have had their work affected due to stress from bullying (Clark & Ahten, 2011)

- Lost productivity resulted in $11,581 per nurse annually (American Nurses Association [ANA], 2015)
- The estimated cost of replacing one specialty nurse (ICU, ER, OR) can exceed $145,000 (Becher & Visovsky, 2012, p. 211)
- It is estimated that productive loss from bullying is 536 hours per nurse, per year. Consider how this affects a health care facility where multiple nurses are bullied
- The estimated cost of replacing one medical–surgical nurse can exceed $92,000 (Christie & Jones, 2014)
- Sixty-six percent of bullied employees admitted to a decline in work performance (Hunt & Zopito, 2012, p. 366)
- Twenty-seven percent of emergency room (ER) nurses reported being bullied (Chipps & McRury, 2012, p. 95)
- Twenty-eight percent of employees lost time at work in order to avoid a bully or those who are uncivil (Hutton & Gates, 2008, p. 169)
- The average age of a bullied nurse is 50 (Castronovo et al., 2016, p. 209)
- The average number of years of experience in nursing of a bullied nurse is 20 (Castronovo et al., 2016, p. 209)
- The financial cost of workplace violence has been estimated to be $400 million a year (Hutton & Gates, 2008)
- Several studies estimate that about a third of all novice nurses who experience workplace bullying in their first position plan to leave (Peggy Berry, 80). Fifty-seven percent leave by the second year (Johnson, 2009, p. 84)
- In 2004, the Institute for Safe Medication Practices conducted a survey showing 7% of nurses reported that they were involved in a medication error within the past year as a result of intimidation in the workplace (Castronovo et al., 2016, p. 210)
- In 2011, an Emergency Department Violence Surveillance Study found that 7,200 ER nurses stated that they were victims of physical or verbal abuse, but they never filed a complaint (Larson, 2013)

- Nurses who are bullied are less likely to seek help and ask questions, potentially leading to errors and substandard patient care (Flateau-Lux & Gravel, 2014, p. 227)

HOW TO FIX THE BULLYING PROBLEM

Many attempts to fix the bullying problem have been proposed by professional organizations in response to the results of studies. It seems that relying on only one method (e.g., educating staff that it is not appropriate to bully, or coaching nurses in how to react to bullying during team-building sessions) is not effective. Establishing and enforcing a zero-tolerance policy, goes beyond what the current literature suggests; it was also not supported until the ANA's position statement, published in 2015. Many laws have been proposed, including the "Healthy Workplace Bill," but never enacted.

Fast Facts in a Nutshell

The most cited reason nurses give for leaving their job is bullying.

References

American Nurses Association. (2015). *Incivility, bullying, and workplace violence*. Washington, DC: Author. Retrieved from http://www.nursingworld.org/MainMenuCategories/WorkplaceSafety/Healthy-Nurse/bullyingworkplaceviolence/Incivility-Bullying-and-Workplace-Violence.html

Becher, J., & Visovsky, C. (2012). Horizontal violence in nursing. *MEDSURG Nursing*, *21*(4), 210–232.

Castronovo, M. A., Pullizzi, A., & Evans, S. (2016). Nurse bullying: A review and a proposed solution. *Nursing Outlook*, *64*, 208–214.

Chipps, E. M., & McRury, M. (2012). The development of an educational intervention to address workplace bullying. *Journal for Nurses in Staff Development, 28*(3), 94–98.

Christie, W., & Jones, S. (2014). Lateral violence in nursing and the theory of the nurse as wounded healer. *Online Journal of Issues in Nursing, 19*(1). Retrieved from http://www.nursingworld.org

Clark, C. M., & Ahten, S. M. (2011, August). Nurses: Resetting the civility conversation. *MedScape Nurses*. Retrieved from http://www.medscape.com/viewarticle/748104

Flateau-Lux, L. R., & Gravel, G. (2014). Put a stop to bullying new nurses. *Home Healthcare Nurse, 32*(4), 225–229.

Hunt, C., & Zopito, A., M. (2012). Incivility in the practice environment: A perspective from clinical nursing teachers. *Nurse Education in Practice, 12*, 366–370.

Hutton, S., & Gates, D. (2008). Workplace incivility and productivity losses among direct care staff. *Workplace Health & Safety, 56*(4), 168–175.

Johnson, S. L. (2009). Workplace bullying: Concerns for nurse leaders. *The Journal of Nursing Administration, 39*(2), 84–90.

Larson, J. (2013). Nurse bullying: An ongoing problem in the health care workplace. Retrieved from http://www.workplacebullying.org

7

Bullying and the Nurse: Effects, Resolution, and Healing

Nurses very often do not report that they have been victims of bullying. "Victims of bullying generally report that using formal and informal organizational channels to bring about an end to bullying was emotionally draining, time-consuming, and often futile" (Johnson & Rea, 2009, p. 88). Nurses often feel that their only recourse and the only end to their treatment is to leave their job or the profession altogether. On the way out of the facility, they very often suggest to their fellow nurses that they just leave. By leaving, however, nurses miss the opportunity to effect a change, but they must consider what is best for their health.

After reading the chapter, the reader will be able to:

- List two outward signs that a nurse is being bullied
- List five mental and physical effects on the nurse who is bullied
- Describe two ways to cope with being bullied
- List five steps that will break the chain of bullying
- Describe how to heal a "walking wounded" nurse

THE EFFECTS OF BULLYING ON THE INDIVIDUAL NURSE

The effects of bullying on the nurse are both physical and psychological. The victim, often silent because of the fear of retaliation or potential loss of job, contains his or her anger. The victim then suffers the physical effects from long-term suppressed feelings of anger.

Fast Facts in a Nutshell

A nurse who is bullied loses sight of his or her reason for being a nurse, and this can be viewed as the greatest loss of all.

Among many signs and symptoms, nurses who are bullied feel:

- Decreased job satisfaction
- Decreased support from their employer or health care organization
- Reduction in self-confidence and self-esteem
- Disillusionment with nursing (Hurley, 2006, p. 70); loss of viewing self as a person capable of being a nurse—someone who can no longer be caring, supportive, sympathetic, or empathetic

"Forty-five percent of people targeted by a bully experience stress-related health problems including debilitating anxiety, panic attacks, and clinical depression (39%)" (Heathfield, 2016). As a nurse, you are aware that stress-related disease can kill you, so put your health first. Other effects on physical and mental health include the following:

- Increased anxiety
- Fear
- Anger
- Sadness
- Depression
- Frustration
- Nervousness
- Embarrassment
- Emotional distress
- Strained personal relationships (family, friends)
- Psychosomatic distress
- Mistrust
- Fatigue
- Headaches
- Eating disorders
- Angina
- Burnout
- Substance abuse
- Posttraumatic stress disorder (PTSD)-related symptoms
- Eating disorders
- Cardiovascular disease
- Increased blood pressure
- Suicidal ideation

HOW TO COPE

Nursing is a stressful occupation. Having to deal with the stress of a profession while also being bullied places a great toll on the physical and mental well-being of the nurse. To cope with bullying, nurses

- Should not attempt to personalize an attack
- May find it helpful to discuss the situation and their feelings with a trusted friend, coworker, or educator
    - Speaking about the experience helps the victim verify that the actions of the perpetrator were actually bullying

- Should seek counseling as soon as possible after the event to decrease emotional trauma
  - Counseling should include assertiveness training so that the victim can learn to deal with situations of bullying in the future
- May also use journaling as a method in dealing with bullying
  - It provides a way for the nurse to document events (e.g., dates, times, witnesses and all notes, e-mails, and texts that may have been produced)
  - It provides an emotional outlet for the distress caused by bullying
- Should participate in stress reduction activities, such as enjoying time with family and friends, surrounding themselves with positive people, exercising, eating healthy, enjoying music, taking breaks, talking to a trusted friend, getting fresh air, participating in hobbies, and making physical and mental health a priority

YOU ARE BEING BULLIED . . . WHAT SHOULD YOU DO?

Everyone who has ever been bullied asks what he or she can do to either prevent it from occurring or to prevent it from reoccurring. Our mothers' answer "just ignore it and it will stop" does not work, and it may also, as we have reviewed, place patients' lives in danger. One study found that 50% of bullying incidents were not reported because victims or witnesses feared retaliation, including being fired (Castronovo, Pullizzi, & Evans, 2016, p. 210). Another study reported that 74% of victims were dissatisfied with the outcome when they tried to take action against the bully (Castronovo et al., 2016, p. 210). Also refer to Chapter 9 for other anti-bullying techniques as well as this resource (www.kickbully.com). It is an unfortunate reality that if you go against the bully, you should be prepared to go alone. If you have close friends or colleagues, they may not help you because they are trying to preserve their own careers. Also be prepared that human resources and upper-level management will not assist either. Be prepared financially as well as with another job in the offing should fighting the bully not go as you hoped. Appropriate steps to take if you are being bullied include the following and more can be found at the aforementioned website:

- Do not ignore or excuse the behavior
- Set limits on what you will tolerate from the bully. If the bully crosses the line, then let him or her know that he or she must stop the behavior. It may be helpful to rehearse what you will say to a friend (role-play) so that you are comfortable with what you want to say and prepared for when the time occurs.
- Be aware of unit or facility policies and procedures in dealing with hostile behavior and bullying
- Try not to be afraid; fear will cause you to not take action against the behavior
- Begin by attempting to come to a resolution between you and the bully
  - Immediately or very soon after the event, the bullying actions should be addressed
  - If needed, create mental space between you and the bully by walking away from the situation. This is done when immediate resolution is not possible
  - If possible and you are not in immediate danger, tell the person who is bullying you how his or her actions are making you feel
  - If needed, elicit the help of an objective third party
  - Do not argue but focus on the facts that occurred. Tell the bully exactly what behavior you see him or her exhibiting and what you want stopped
  - Insist that all bullying behavior stop—be specific about the behavior you wished stopped

  - Do not state how the behavior made you feel—how his or her behavior is impacting the care of your patients or work overall
  - Do not attempt to reason with the bully or to attempt to have the bully understand how he or she is making you feel
  - Tell the bully exactly what behavior you will not tolerate in the future
  - If the bully crosses the line and violates your set limit, then you must consider how to fight the bully or reporting (see Chapter 9)
- Be aware that if you speak up and attempt to defend yourself, it may encourage the bully to continue the behavior
- Give the action a name, call a bully a "bully" and what he or she is demonstrating is bullying or uncivil behavior, and get it out in the open
- Document. Include the date, time, location, and those involved. Give specific details of what occurred, including how you attempted to stop the behavior. The fact that patient care is being impacted will be important to management.
- Keep copies of all e-mails and other documentation sent to you by the bully
- Notify nursing leadership following the proper chain of command. If you skip the first steps and report bullying directly to management, they will more likely ask you to communicate with the perpetrator first and attempt to resolve the situation on your own.
- If the charge nurse, nurse manager, or director of nursing is the bully, report the incident to human resources and ask for assistance.
- Ask for help in dealing with the bully. Refer to facility policies regarding what help is available for employees dealing with workplace bullying and violence.
- Be aware of what actions warrant notification of the police. These include public slander, physical abuse, or other

criminal actions. When in doubt, always notify your human resources department.

- If you feel uncomfortable, immediately address the bully's behavior. It is thought that some bullies are unaware that their actions and words are causing distress.
- Speak about bullying at staff meetings—bring it out in the open
- Speak to human resources (or similar department) in your facility about how to deal with the situation.
- Document occurrences of bullying that you personally witness
- Note and document if the person bullying you also bullies others. Be sure that all others are documenting as well. More proof of bullying by multiple parties will have more of an impact
- Be aware of your own behaviors
- Do not share your documentation with anyone
- Take care of you! Work stress reduction into your daily schedule.
- Do not take matters into your own hands and retaliate against the perpetrator
- See professional counseling if needed

Fast Facts in a Nutshell

"Interestingly, five nurses in one study who spoke out against horizontal violence reported positive outcomes from 'standing up for myself'" (Hurley, 2006, p. 70).

If dealing directly with the bully places you in danger or is not a possibility, then take the following steps:

- Walk away from the situation and find a safe area if necessary.
- Seek out someone whom you trust when reporting the incident.

STEPS TO TAKE TO BREAK THE CHAIN OF BULLYING

As previously stated, bullying behavior is cyclical. Aggressive behavior by another nurse triggers anger in a colleague. Then anger triggers abrasive behavior in another colleague and the behavior is reinforced because it is ignored. How can the cycle be broken?

- Be attentive and actively listen to those with whom you interact, including patients.
- In all communications with staff, patients, and significant others, be open, honest, and respectful.
- Be aware of self. Are you exhibiting bullying or uncivil behaviors? Are you supporting the bullying actions of others? Are you involved in healthy personal relationships with your coworkers? Are you a member of a clique that discriminates against others?
- Be accountable for your behavior. Hold others accountable for theirs.
- Do not be afraid to use the term *bully* when referring to the behavior of others—the longer that nurses attempt to hide its existence, the longer it will continue.
- When you are listening, restate what you heard to ensure what you heard was correct.
- Follow the Golden Rule: "Do unto others as you would have them do unto you." In other words, treat everyone (patient, family member, fellow staff, administrator) the way you would like to be treated.
- Empathy and compassion are therapeutic techniques that should not be confined to just patients; they should be used with all with whom we interact including fellow staff.
- Do not assume that everyone is "against you" or that every comment is meant to hurt you.
- Be civil with all with whom you interact. Use kindness, consideration, and courtesy.

- Act in a professional manner in all your interactions. This also means to be answerable for errors that occur or work/care that was not completed.
- Model professional behavior.
- Be willing to report bullying and incivility.
- Always remember yourself in the role of a student, novice nurse, or new employee. Recall what it was like to be that person and treat him or her how you would have liked to have been treated.
- Resist the temptation to gossip.
- Participate in conflict resolution, diversity, and effective communication-learning opportunities, both in-house and at outside offerings.
- Befriend new staff members; welcome them to the unit, and introduce them to fellow staff members and other personnel.
- Speak kindly to those who are bullied, and be supportive.
- Do not assume that a victim of bullying requires your assistance; ask first.
- Encourage your fellow staff members to work as a team in order to eliminate abusive behavior.
- Become a mentor for new staff.
- Be the person who begins the change of the unit/facility culture. Participate in facility committees and share your experiences and successes.
- Encourage victims to speak up and stand up for themselves. Be supportive of their actions.

Fast Facts in a Nutshell

Many nurses do not feel it is either possible or within their scope of responsibility to stop bullying.

NURSES DO NOT LET NURSES BULLY

Nurses everywhere state that they have been "forced" to witness the mistreatment and bullying of their colleagues. They note the behaviors of the perpetrator, the witnesses, and the victim. They also state that even though they saw the fear and anxiety their colleagues were experiencing, they did not step in to stop the bully because they feared the bully and they feared losing their jobs. Not only does the victim of bullying suffer the effects of the behavior, the witness does as well, including symptoms of decreased self-esteem, depression, and anger. Nurses who witness bullying should do the following:

- Be aware of unit/facility policies and procedures regarding bullying.
- Call for help following facility guidelines—the incident should be brought immediately to the attention of the appropriate individual.
- Not support the bullying actions of others.
- Support the victim by providing witness statements, documentation, and other called-for actions when appropriate to be taken, such as in a legal proceeding.
- Not let an incident of bullying occur while present, or act to stop it and/or report it as per unit/facility policy if it occurs.
- Not join in on a gossip session, or with a group that is teasing or laughing at another nurse. Refuse to spread gossip.
- Support a fellow nurse who has been the victim of bullying. Provide emotional support, validation, and assistance with documentation.

SIGNS AND SYMPTOMS

During the normal stress that is part of the health care system, fellow staff members may not recognize when a fellow nurse is being bullied. There are common signs and symptoms to be aware of and these include the following:

- Appearing exhausted
- Taking "mental health days"
- Verbalization of depression
- Frequent absenteeism
- Frequent complaints of (somatic) illness and physical distress
- Verbalization of thoughts of suicide
- Verbalization of the feeling of "burnout"
- Complaint of headaches
- Eating disorders
- Depression

HEALING THE "WALKING WOUNDED NURSE"

As mentioned in Chapter 4, in order for a nurse to become a "wounded healer," he or she must recognize and overcome the pain and suffering of the past. According to Conti-O'Hare who put forth this theory in 2002, nurses must first be able to recognize what occurred (Christie & Jones, 2014). They need ask themselves:

- What happened to cause the pain/trauma?
- What if anything could have been changed?
- How should it have been handled differently?

Once nurses have recognized the cause of the trauma and pain, they must then begin the process of transforming the incident into a manageable aspect of their lives. They do this by asking themselves:

- What can I learn from this incident?
- Has the incident affected me or the people about whom I care?
- Can this incident be used by me to make my life better?

After successfully recognizing the incident and transforming it, nurses must then transcend the incident. This means that they use what they have learned from moving through the steps in order to assist others around them, including patients and colleagues dealing with their pain and trauma. The nurse is able to say, if not aloud, then to self in her or his actions and care: "I understand your pain" and "How can I make things better for you?" The nurse must successfully move through all three steps in order to become a "wounded healer" who has the ability to empathize with another person. According to Conti-O'Hare, "professional relationships improve, resulting in a more positive work environment, and overall patient care is optimized" (Christie & Jones, 2014). If the nurse suffers another traumatic incident, he or she must move through the steps again.

ZERO TOLERANCE MAY NOT BE THE ANSWER

Many nurse theorists, authors, and even the American Nurses Association (ANA) state that only zero tolerance is the answer to stop bullying. Although this is an aspect of stopping the behavior, it must be undertaken *along with* other policies. Those in leadership should do the following:

- Adopt the core values of staff empowerment, effective communication, mutual collaboration, and learning.
- Model professional behavior.
- Celebrate educational and professional achievements.
- Celebrate and value the uniqueness of each staff member.
- Remind staff of what it was like to be new, when a new nurse employee or novice nurse begins work on the unit; Encourage them to share their stories with the new nurse.
- Ensure that your facility provides an adequate orientation for new staff; ensure that staff development guidelines regarding orientation are followed.
- Utilize preceptors that support anti-bullying policies: who are supportive of new staff: who will intervene when

they witness bullying behavior (thus breaking the cycle—the new nurse will observe anti-bullying behavior and "pass it on").

- Educate all staff on how to report bullying incidents and ensure them that acts of reprisal will not be tolerated.
- Be mindful of the possibility of increased bullying since it has been found that when a facility undergoes organizational restructuring or other change, it allows bullies to flourish as they take advantage of their authority to further their careers.
- Ensure that the facility has implemented evidence-based interventions that staff can utilize to prevent and respond to bullying. Included should be documenting incidents and actions to take during an incident. Ensure that staff are educated regarding the interventions.
- Staff evaluations should reflect negatively on those who demonstrate bullying behavior.

Zero-tolerance policies should include methods of reporting and enforcement. There should also be mentioned methods of measurement in order to ensure that the policy and all other measures have created the necessary changes.

Fast Facts in a Nutshell

"Most experts agree that it takes 2 to 5 years for an organization to change its culture" (Harris, 2013).

References

Castronovo, M. A., Pullizzi, A., & Evans, S. (2016). Nurse bullying: A review and a proposed solution. *Nursing Outlook, 64*, 208–214.

Christie, W., & Jones, S. (2014). Lateral violence in nursing and the theory of the nurse as wounded healer. *Online Journal of Issues in Nursing, 19*, 1–11. Retrieved from http://www.nursingworld.org

Harris, C. (2013). Incivility in nursing. *Nursing Bulletin—Official Publication of the North Carolina Board of Nursing.* Retrieved from http://www.ncbon.com/dcp/i/nursing-education-continuing-education-board-sponsored-bulletin-offerings-incivility-in-nursing

Heathfield, S. M. (2016). How to deal with a bully at work: Don't be an easy target for a bully. Retrieved from https://www.thebalance.com/how-to-deal-with-a-bully-at-work-1917901

Hurley, J. E. (2006, September). Nurse-to-nurse horizontal violence: Recognizing it and preventing it. *National Student Nurses' Association Imprint, 53*(4), 68–71.

Johnson, S. L., & Rea, R. E. (2009). Workplace bullying concerns for nurse leaders. *Journal of Nursing Administration, 39*(2), 84–90.

8

The Responsibilities of Nursing Leadership and the Employer

To the outside world, those who are in leadership positions in nursing are placed there because, obviously, they are the best qualified for the position. They are viewed as having had many years of education and training to prepare them for their prospective positions. We in nursing, however, know of a different aspect of nurse leadership. Many nurse leaders are viewed as "the next in line," that a given position was not wanted by other nurses or someone in a position of authority allowed someone to take a higher position. Those in leadership, as nurses are aware, know very little regarding leading and being in charge. They treat others as they have been treated—if they were bullied, then they themselves become bullies because they are now in a position of power.

After reading this chapter, the reader will be able to:

- List five things nurse leaders should be aware of when monitoring their unit for bullying

(*continued*)

- Describe five actions nurse leaders or those in management can do to control and eliminate bullying
- List five steps in a bullying investigation
- Define "empowerment"
- Define "silence as acceptance"

LEADERSHIP STANDARDS

Several bullying studies have noted that bullying is more pervasive in health care facilities where employees feel that bullying is tolerated, that those who bully are indirectly rewarded (pay raises, job promotions), and that the behavior has approval from management simply because it is tolerated. In fact, "up to 81% of employers are perceived as doing nothing and resisting taking action when targets of bullying fill out a survey. In the general public, only 44.8% perceive the employers as doing nothing" (Heathfield, 2016).

In 2009, The Joint Commission set forth leadership standards for those facilities that sought or held accreditation. These standards are:

- Establishing a code of conduct that addresses adverse behaviors
- Promoting a nonpunitive forum that allows the reporting of adverse behaviors
- Creating a disciplinary process for those employees who bully their colleagues

SILENT ACCEPTANCE

When nurse leaders or facility administrators are silent in the face of bullying and uncivil behavior, they unknowingly (or knowingly) condone the behavior. If staff observe that leadership is tolerating bullying and uncivil behavior, then they feel that they have no recourse and no one to whom to turn for help; staff do not feel that they can safely report being bullied. Parenthetically, the bully sees this silence as acceptance and continues the behavior. Those who bully have a supportive atmosphere to continue terrorizing their colleagues. They are supported as they move ahead in their careers and to various job postings within the facility, thus reinforcing the fact that a bully is very often in a leadership position. This is compounded if the bully leader is also productive and meets the goals of the facility. Very often, others in leadership positions may not approve of the behavior or even be aware that it is occurring but the staff understand that silence is acceptance.

Many nurse leaders and administrators feel that they are unable to deal with bullying and incivility. Unfortunately, many see their staff only as employees to get a job done. Their presence or absence affects patient care and the bottom line. It does not matter to them what is affecting the nurse/employee, but only that the victim's behavior is affecting the unit. The victim is not seen as a person with rights. As has been noted in the previous chapters, the cycle of bullying and victimhood is perpetuated when one who has been bullied feels powerless and remains silent.

Constant monitoring by those in nursing administration should take place in order to be aware of any instance of bullying or incivility. Policy and procedure intervention is appropriate when an incident takes place; however, the key to stopping bullying is to be aware of what causes the behavior, knowing who is vulnerable, and preventing the behavior. The staff member who is experiencing bullying should not assume, however, that nursing leadership is aware that a problem exists, and should also not assume that the behavior has already been reported, but not acted upon.

For what should the nurse leader be on the lookout when monitoring the staff?

- Nonverbal behaviors such as facial expressions in response to comments from the victim to a fellow nurse
- Failure to respect the privacy of another nurse

- Speaking or complaining behind another nurse's back instead of confronting conflict directly
- Betraying confidences
- Not taking responsibility for actions and blaming others in a bad situation
- The existence of cliques that exclude others
- In-fighting among the staff
- A staff member purposely being set up for failure on the unit (increased patient ratio with high acuity; not helping another nurse; watching a nurse struggle while attempting care for the patient)
- Withholding patient care information
- Snide or rude remarks or abrupt answers to questions

LEADERS TAKE ACTION

It is a well-known fact among staff nurses that many of those in nursing management do not belong there and that many people in the hospital administration or ownership of health care facilities do not belong there either. Whether it is a lack of education in organizational leadership or a lack of experience, many nurse managers and administrators have difficulty dealing with day-to-day issues, let alone bullying on a unit or in a facility.

Fast Facts in a Nutshell

"Characteristics that contribute to bullying are a rigid, vertical organization structure, informal alliances and hierarchies, imbalance of power, job insecurity, and organizational wide restructuring and downsizing" (Wright & Naresh, 2015, p. 146).

It is also well known that mangers often ignore policies on bullying because they feel that they are ineffective or that bullying itself is not an issue. How can this be rectified? What can those in administration and nursing leadership do to prevent and eliminate bullying?

- Those in nursing leadership and health care administration should first be educated regarding bullying, incivility, and workplace violence—education regarding bullying prevention should be evidence based.
  - Facility staff development should provide ongoing education for current staff and within new staff orientation—all staff, including leadership, should fully understand the impact of bullying and incivility in nursing.
  - Ongoing education should also include how to "practice emotional intelligence, crucial conversations . . . sensitivity training . . . and team communications" (Wright & Naresh, 2015, p. 146).
  - During orientation and throughout an employee's tenure, there should be education for staff on recognizing bullying behaviors and coaching of staff to create and enforce skills of collaboration, communication, and acceptance of differences (Wright & Naresh, 2015, p. 146).
- Be aware of their own actions and words. Are they bullies? All the mission statements and zero-tolerance policies in the world will not be effective if nursing leaders and administrators do not model the behavior they wish to see in their staff.
- Name the action of the perpetrator as "bullying" or "horizontal violence," and get it out in the open and freely expressed, not hidden.
- Take the opportunity of staff meetings to speak on the issue. Use it as a chance to educate the staff and make them aware that no incidents will be tolerated. Encourage staff to speak up about occurrences where they have witnessed or been victims of bullying.
- Ensure that there are facility policies and procedures in place to deal with bullying and incivility. If they are not in place, be part of a team that creates them, following

American Nurses Association (ANA) and other authoritarian guidelines.

- Staff may not report bullying because they fear being reprimanded or that the system will not work.
- Reporting mechanisms must be clearly defined and easy to follow—reporting should not directly be to the direct line supervisor, as he or she may be the bully.
- Staff must be able to trust those to whom they are reporting an incident and trust the system designed to assist them.
- Consider a bullying "hot line" or other such mechanism that is convenient for staff on all shifts.
- Human resources, or similar department, need to house and conduct its own grievance procedure and investigation mechanisms. As stated, bullies may have alliances that help to subvert policies, and either minimize or ignore a report of bullying. No one involved in a bullying incident should ever be involved in the investigation as well. Consider an ombudsperson position within the facility, a third person to whom the nurses can turn and report bullying without fear of retaliation.

- Policies should reflect codes of conduct. These documents should be accessible to all staff, given to all staff at orientation, and revisited/reviewed yearly. This should be documented in an employee's file.
- Be fully committed to eradicating bullying from a unit/facility. Avoid, however, just moving a bully from unit to unit in order to avoid removing a productive employee. This sends a signal to other bullies that their behavior is condoned. Alliances among bullies exist and victims may find themselves the target of abuse again.
- Leadership should be required to create and enforce a culture of respect within the facility and among all health care workers.

- *Immediately* acknowledge staff concerns and complaints—however, endeavor to act only on sincere, accurate information.
- Actively listen to concerns of staff.
- Be on the lookout for the formation or existence of cliques. Promote trust among the staff and a collegial atmosphere.
- If a unit self-governs, monitor that decisions made are fair, accountable, and responsible.
- Utilize appropriate negotiation strategies when dealing with issues on the unit—never have confrontation; consider compromise.
- Communicate timely information concerning bullying on the unit or within the facility.
- Openly question staff regarding their opinions on unit/facility issues and patient care needs. Be open and honest with staff about what can be "fixed" within the unit/facility and what cannot and how staff can assist. If you do not know the answer to a question, state that you do not know but that you will find the answer and then do so.
- Be supportive of all staff.
- Ensure that those who precept new nurses or students are educated in how to properly precept. Do not pick an RN to be a preceptor because it is his or her "turn," but rather because he or she wants to assist new nurses. Ensure that those who precept are properly compensated.
- Be fair and consistent in dealings with all staff. What policy for one is policy for all, and this includes staffing levels, scheduling, and assignments.
- Be aware, at all times, of unit culture—has anything altered the emotional atmosphere of the unit? Be aware of the staff morale. Observe both verbal and nonverbal behavior.
- Be sympathetic and empathetic.
- Be a champion of open communication. However, encourage and enforce the use of formal communication and

follow proper channels of communication for all staff. The door cannot be open to one and closed to another.

- Be supportive of nurses returning for their degrees or advancing on clinical ladders or of support staff advancing their education. Ensure that all staff are allowed time off the unit for staff education and in-services.
- Encourage and allow staff to participate in extracurricular activities that decrease stress and promote relaxation.
- Do not blame the targets of the bully and let them know that the incident(s) are not their fault.
- Do not assume that the victim requires your assistance. If you witness bullying, ask the victim if he or she requires assistance.
- Ensure that your staff are accountable for their actions.
- Encourage assertiveness, discourage aggression. Provide and encourage staff to participate in conflict management and self-defense training.
- Ensure that staffing levels are adequate and safe.
- Make victims aware of employee assistance programs available to them.
- When an employee leaves a unit, conduct an exit after he or she leaves. This will provide information as to what led the staff person to leave and what factors may need to be corrected.

BULLYING INVESTIGATION

Those in leadership will be called upon to investigate the incident of bullying. This should be conducted by those who do not have regular contact or supervision of the employees involved. However, a unit manager may be asked to conduct an investigation and this should be done as quickly as possible after it is reported or witnessed. The nurse leader should:

- Know unit/facility policies regarding bullying and horizontal violence and be prepared to enforce them and initiate disciplinary action if necessary

- Immediately and objectively question all witnesses in an open manner and without blame
- Not assume how an incident occurred without fully investigating the facts
- Document findings following unit/facility protocol
- Report findings immediately as per protocol
- Discipline offenders as per protocol (staff evaluations should reflect the behavior of the perpetrator)
- Provide information on counseling for victims
- Commit to an open-door policy in dealing with all staff and transparency in decision making
- Follow up on how/why the incident took place and how to prevent it from occurring

AS A WHOLE

The facility should utilize the staff to assist it in developing policies and procedures to combat bullying and horizontal violence. Following are some actions unit and facility focus groups can consider:

- Unit and facility focus groups can enable staff to identify areas of improvement and collaborate on ideas to improve communication.
- Focus groups could also study and discuss ways to decrease errors, improve quality of care, decrease nurse turnover, and improve productivity (Becher & Visovsky, 2012, p. 212).
- Lack of support, poor teamwork, respectful behavior, and micromanagement of employees could also be addressed within the focus groups (Becher & Visovsky, 2012, p. 212). These issues, if left unaddressed, often lead to horizontal violence.

EMPOWERMENT

"Empowerment" is not just a 1990s buzzword. Over the years, the definition of empowerment, however, has been lost. Empowerment means that another person has been "given the power" by another person to make decisions, competent choices, and to act with authority, knowledge, and experience (Bradbury-Jones, Sambrook, & Irvine, 2007, p. 343). Nurses who feel that they are autonomous, have a say in the day-to-day workings of a unit, and share in hospital governance councils, unit-based councils, and open communication between staff and management are successful in combating bullying. They allow other nurses to feel valued and important (because they are!). Empowerment is "correlated inversely with workplace incivility and supervisor incivility in the general nursing population . . . as well as bullying among new graduates. . . . acts of incivility and bullying are attempts to take power from others; therefore, structural empowerment is related to lower levels of incivility, bullying and horizontal violence" (Lachman, 2015).

Further exploration of these issues appears in Chapter 17, which presents case studies relating to bullying in nursing administration.

References

Becher, J., & Visovsky, C. (2012). Horizontal violence in nursing. *MEDSURG Nursing*, *21*(4), 210–232.

Bradbury-Jones, C., Sambrook, S., & Irvine, F. (2007). The meaning of empowerment for nursing students: A critical incident study. *Journal of Advanced Nursing*, *59*(4), 342–351.

Heathfield, S. M. (2016). How to deal with a bully at work: Don't be an easy target for a bully. Retrieved from https://www.thebalance.com/how-to-deal-with-a-bully-at-work-1917901

Lachman, V. D. (2015). Ethical issues in the disruptive behaviors of incivility, bullying, and horizontal/lateral violence. *Urology Nurse*, *35*(1), 39–42.

Wright, W., & Naresh, K. (2015). Bullying among nursing staff: Relationship with psychological/behavioral responses of nurses and medical errors. *Health Care Management Review*, *40*(2), 139–147.

9

Resisting a Bully

Specific techniques to deal with a bully in the workplace are described in this chapter. Ironically, these techniques were *not* found in any nursing journal, but on websites and in business journals. This is another indicator of how far health care lags behind other fields when dealing with bullying behavior of staff or leadership. Other tools to assist nurses in assessing and dealing with a bully can be found online at www.kickbully.com.

After reading this chapter, the reader will be able to:

- Explain how to determine if you are being bullied
- List five steps that will help you be prepared to combat a bully
- List how to mentally prepare yourself to confront a bully
- List the stages of confronting a bully
- Describe techniques used in each of the three types of bullies

PREPARE YOURSELF TO RESPOND

Usually the first instinct when confronted with a bully is to fight back. You visualize how you will be triumphant against the bully, everything at work will be perfect, and everyone will get along. To be effective in the confrontation, you need to take your time and prepare yourself both mentally and with a backup plan for another employment should the situation not resolve. To be prepared to fight against bullying, you should keep in mind the following points:

- Depending on leadership's feelings about bullying, and if the bully *is* in leadership, prepare for a long battle.
- Have a positive outlook that all including the bully will see—be calm and maintain your sense of humor; by not showing others that you are bothered by the bully, you become less of a target.
- Expect to go into battle alone. Your friends and colleagues may not wish to help you because they are concerned with their own jobs and careers.
- Always assume that human resources, until proved otherwise, will be on the side of the bully. This is one of the situations that health care must change because it has led to the continuation of bullying over decades.
- Be prepared to be moved to another unit, another facility, or fired outright. Do not begin the battle until you have another position to which to go. Be aware of your current financial situation. Can you afford to be fired?
- Begin planning how to best approach the bully. If you cannot afford to leave your current job or while you are actively searching another job, use a more conservative approach.
- Always keep in mind the type of bully with whom you are dealing; you must control the situation because, in a case against a bully who is a manipulator, by being emotional you are giving him or her more ammunition to use against you.

MENTAL PREPARATION

The bully is excellent at keeping you mentally off your feet. Each day, each minute, you may find him or her saying and doing things that keep you wondering whether he or she truly is a bully or you are the one with the problem. One day the bully is telling you how great you are and the next day the bully is screaming at you in front of patients and colleagues. Be aware that the bully is manipulating you and be calm. The more upset you become because of this, the more difficult it will be for you to control your emotions. Be clear about the fight that you are about to undergo and understand that it may be a long fight and that it may not end with eliminating the bully and you remaining on the unit, but it will end and it will end with you being in a better place and away from the bully and the allies.

The steps for preparing mentally include the following:

- Vent your anger, to yourself and not within earshot of the bully. Vent to a friend who is not a colleague.
- Change your outlook.
  - Identify what is *really* going on within the unit and the health care facility as a whole.
  - Understand the roles each one plays, the code of conduct, relationships between leaders, who has perceived and actual power.
  - Is the system undergoing any changes (takeovers, mergers, or is it failing)?
  - Has anyone ever been fired for bullying?
  - Is there currently a bully who has the support of human resources or leadership? Has anyone ever complained about this bully? What happened to them (the bully *and* the victim)?
  - Has the facility recently adopted "zero tolerance" policies and all the policies and changes that need to accompany this outlook toward bullies?
  - Be fully aware of what will happen if you lose the battle against the bully—job loss, loss of friends, feelings of incompetence, sadness, anger, and frustration.

    - Be fully aware of what will happen if you win the battle against the bully—is your job worth the effort it will take? Will you be happy staying on your unit or within the facility? Would it be better to find another job or continue your education?
    - Know the alternatives to combating the bully. Can you avoid the bully by transferring to another unit or another part of the health care system? Should you quit and find another job?
    - Face your fears about leaving. Will it be difficult to find a new job? Has the bully already convinced you that you are a poor nurse and unable to find work at another facility?
    - Understand what will happen if you do nothing. Will your health or personal life be affected if you stay?
- Prepare yourself for the unpleasant happening and you will not be disappointed. Be prepared to face the cruelty of the bully, the lack of support from colleagues and friends, and the praise and honor given to the bully even when you thought he or she would be fired.
    - The bully will become even nastier the more you fight him or her. The manipulation will continue and become worse. Expect to be slandered and lied about. Your reputation may be ruined.
    - Your fellow staff will be intimidated into not supporting you. They may be unaware of what the bully is doing to you but believe the management propaganda that it is a "personality conflict" between you and the bully. Expect fellow staff to betray you and talk behind your back, and you may become isolated. In time, the same staff who did not support you in your fight may be bullied as well, but it will be too late for you to help them. You may also not receive support from your significant others unless they themselves have experienced bullying.
    - Expect the battle against the bully to be long and nasty—you may become overwhelmed and frustrated.

  - Know your ultimate goal and be open to opportunities that become evident along the way including personal growth.
- Your commitment must meet and exceed that of the bully.

Fast Facts in a Nutshell

Once you become a target of a bully, there is a chance that you will lose your job. Therefore, you must carefully weigh the choice between staying at or leaving your job if you are being bullied and your workplace does not recognize and assist the victims of bullying.

THE STAGES OF COMBATING A WORKPLACE BULLY

Once you have determined that you will combat the bully, you must assess the bully and determine the type of bully he or she is and the type of methods you will use.

- First, determine that the person is, indeed, a bully and not just someone who may be ineffectively coping with some life experience outside of work. Does the bully meet the definitions set forth in Chapters 2 and 4?
- Determine the type of bully he or she is (as discussed later) and also attempt a friendly conversation with the bully, noting his or her words and behavior. Question coworkers by stating a typical behavior the bully displays and look for reactions from your colleagues (nodding, eye-rolling, and shared stories). Ask if anyone has ever tried to go against the bully and what happened.
- Prepare to fight by reviewing the different techniques listed here and in the resources provided at the end of this chapter.
- Fight back. Prior to this step is the last chance to change your mind. Quit or fight. Make sure you have reviewed all the steps and clearly know what you desire.

HOW TO HANDLE THE "TYPICAL" BULLY

There is no one "typical" bully. Rather, there are different types of bullies, many of whom do not even recognize that they are bullies. For example, the "nonthreatening" bully may be an overwhelmed coworker or someone who is socially inept. You would deal with him or her differently than the person who is an aggressive bully. If you do not like handling confrontation, but would rather let things go hoping that they will blow over, consider how effective that really is. You become frustrated and angry yourself (remember the cycle of bullying?). The bully may repeat the behavior and the situation deteriorates until you either quit or are fired. Would you not rather solve the situation immediately? Suggested steps in handling a nonthreatening bully include:

- **Ignore the behavior**—This is useful if the behavior is rare. You could say something like "Okay, well, see you later" or "Thank you for letting me know." If the behavior is completely out of character of the person, you could just ask him or her a friendly question unrelated to what he or she just said. Polite conversation disarms the bully.
- **Dismiss the bullying—**If the same person has bullied before, but the behavior is still more of a minor annoyance, then quickly address it with a canned, maybe even snarky, response such as "Give me a break" or "Oh, please" and then change the subject. Contradicting what the nonthreatening bully says also works, especially if the bully is speaking about a coworker. Phrases like "That's not the way it happened" or "That's not true" can be used.
- **Seek to understand the bully**—By utilizing empathy, you change the bully's opinion of you from one of adversary to potential friend. For example, use phrases such as "Why are you so upset over this?" or "I'm sorry you're upset. I can understand how you might see what happened that way."

- **Give a friendly speech**—This helps to control the situation; basically, this technique is therapeutic communication for bullies.
  - Show that you care and are a good listener—restate what the bully is saying and then repeat back what you think you have understood.
  - Show sympathy for his or her particular concern—use phrases such as "You shouldn't have to deal with this" and then state why, from the bully's point of view, you feel that they should not be dealing with what they are dealing.
  - Show sincere appreciation for the person—verbalize what you appreciate about them (hard worker, great at patient care, etc.).
  - Speak to how you will address the situation or help him or her—state specifically how you will help him or her deal with the situation. "I'm going to ____. Is that okay with you?" or "Would you rather that I ____________?"
  - If what you are saying is ignored, then repeat what you will do to assist the bully, but the bully needs to choose how the assistance will take place.
  - If the bully does not choose how you can assist him or her, this conversation at least puts the bully on notice that you will not tolerate being bullied. End the conversation.

Another type of bully is the "consistent bully." This is a bully who consistently causes you problems and with whom the nice approach does not work. Suggested steps in handling a consistent bully include:

- **Just say no**—This is useful when the bully keeps expressing the same unreasonable demands.
  - This technique may or may not be effective, but is should be regarded as the first line of defense. Start by saying "No, I'm sorry, I won't ____________."

    - Repeat this until the bully stops demanding a particular action from you.
    - If the bully will not listen, you may need to be more forceful. This may not work in a situation where you as a staff nurse are bullied by a manager or supervisor.
- **Put the bully off**—This means that instead of leaping directly into an argument with the bully, you use phrases that will delay your response.
    - Use phrases such as "I'll get back to you" or "I need to think it over."
    - Keep repeating the responses until the bully either leaves you alone or you need to go to the next step.
- **Confront the bully privately**—This technique can go either way in its effectiveness. Either the bully will stop or he or she will see it as gaining even more power over you.
    - Choose a neutral, private location.
    - Have a bullet-point list of topics you wish to discuss.
    - Be positive and friendly.
    - State that you are trying to discover how to work better together.
    - If the bully begins to become angry or starts losing control, excuse yourself and state that you would rather wait until he or she is less angry.
    - Always state facts, never how his or her behavior makes you feel. The bully does not care how you feel, which is why he or she is a bully. Use phrases like "I was told you said ______________ about me. Is this true?" or "Can you suggest some things we can do to solve this problem?"
    - After you receive a response, ask follow-up questions to be sure you have all the information you need and to possibly figure out why he or she is bullying you.
    - If the bully has a reasonable suggestion, then agree and end the meeting. However, what usually occurs is that the bully is unable to give any useful suggestions in which case you should proceed to "give a friendly

speech" step as previously mentioned. Start by explaining what you think is the issue from his or her point of view. Then state that it is your intention to find a solution to your issues. Tell the bully how you specifically will resolve the issue and then ask if the bully feels that this resolution is acceptable or ask him or her to choose an alternative resolution.

- End the confrontation and leave the meeting. Know that if you did not resolve the situation, at least the bully is aware that you will no longer tolerate his or her behavior.

Fast Facts in a Nutshell

Bullies prefer to exploit individuals whose responses to their bullying are weak and submissive. Thus, when responding to a bully, "You only need to differentiate yourself. Just gently confront any aggressive behavior that comes your way, and the bully will leave you alone and go find an easier target" (kickbully.com, 2017).

The last type of bully is the "highly aggressive bully" who requires different techniques. Caution is in order when confronting this type of bully to avoid escalating the situation and increasing the bully's retaliation. Suggested steps in handling a highly aggressive bully include:

- **Allow the bully to speak**—Try to find out why he or she is angry or upset with you or a situation. Again, use therapeutic (reflective) statements, such as "You seem angry" or "You seem upset."
- **Question the bully's thinking**—Try to find out why he or she is really concerned by saying something like "What is your real concern?" or "What do you feel the

real problem is?" The bully will usually hold back information though, but you may acquire additional information behind what his or her true motives are for bullying you.

- **Apologize**—This apology is not heartfelt or meant on your part, but after saying it, walk away. For example, "I'm sorry that I bother you so much."
- **Force the bully to make a point**—This involves direct questioning and is a power weapon against the bully. Examples include "What is your point?" or "What do you mean?" or "Is anyone else confused by these comments?" (*Warning*: More forceful comments like these used against a nurse manager may get you fired.)
- **Force the bully to explain his or her behavior**—Use questions such as "Why are you blaming me?" or "What is your problem with me?"
- **Openly criticize the bully**—This step is not recommended as it switches you to the role of the bully if done in front of others. It should be used only if you are saying it in front of an audience that is sympathetic to you or has been bullied as well.
- **Tell the bully that you know what he or she is doing**—This is an open confrontation technique used during a one-to-one confrontation and should be used cautiously. Although the bully will deny his or her behavior, it will send a message that you are on to his or her bullying behavior.
- **Tell the bully to leave you alone**—Again, this is not highly recommended as the bully will feel that he or she has gained power over you.
- **Tell the bully that something is wrong with him or her**—Again, this is not recommended and should be used with caution, but it places the bully on the defensive. Use phrases like, "Are you okay?" or "What's wrong with you?"
- **Use compassion**—State that the bully is really a good person who is exhibiting bad behavior. By recognizing that

there may be a good person underneath the intolerable acts of the bully, you will either change that person's life by understanding his or her behavior or help yourself heal.

NOW WHAT HAPPENS

If the bullying you are dealing with has become so intolerant that it has affected your health and your ability to safely do your job, then it is time to consider either fighting back or leaving. However, be aware of the following:

- If utilizing employee assistance counselors, be wary that they may not hold what is told them in confidence. Also, be leery of any counselor or mental health professional who does not believe your story of victimhood. He or she may try to convince you that you are the reason you are being bullied.
- If you plan to fight back and expose the bully, you should also be prepared to find a new job as the environment of tolerance of bullying within your facility may be slow to change. Leaving may be better for your health, your family, and your career. It should not be viewed as giving up, but rather keeping yourself sane and healthy, but remember "good employers purge bullies, most promote them" (Workplace Bullying Institute, 2017).

Fast Facts in a Nutshell

If you do leave a facility due to bullying, then do so with your head held high. Do not leave without telling your story to all you meet. Do not be ashamed of what you have endured. The trauma of the bullying is intensified in those who remain silent (Workplace Bullying Institute).

References

kickbully.com. (2017). Your guide to fighting workplace bullies. Retrieved from http://www.kickbully.com

Workplace Bullying Institute. (2017). Retrieved from http://www.workplacebullying.org

10

Nurse Bullying and the Law

Jackeline Biddle Shuler

Bullying in a workplace is a complex problem that is not presently prohibited by law. Although workplace bullying is not formally prohibited, there are legal remedies and actions that target bullying conduct and pervasive behaviors that threaten the workplace environment of a nurse. This chapter explores the movement for formal workplace bullying legislation. Nurses can use the protections of existing legal remedies that prohibit bullying behaviors without having to make a claim for bullying. But more importantly, nurses should advocate for legislative changes that would make abusive workplace environments illegal.

After reading this chapter, the reader will be able to:

- Describe the current state of bullying in the nursing workplace
- List legal claims that can arise from bullying in the workplace
- Report bullying conduct in the workplace

(continued)

- Describe recommendations for a model workplace bullying law
- Discuss the nurse's role in legislative advocacy against workplace bullying

SIGNIFICANCE OF BULLYING PREVENTION IN THE NURSING WORK ENVIRONMENT

Registered nurses are required to foster civility and kindness toward others. The American Nurses Association (ANA) *Code of Ethics for Nurses with Interpretive Statements* imposes a moral obligation for registered nurses to acknowledge and take action against behaviors such as bullying (ANA, 2015a). For example, if nurses witness bullying, there is an obligation to report such behaviors in the workplace. Nurses are also expected to serve as role models of professionalism and civility in the workplace. The code of ethics also requires nurses to participate in the development and implementation of policies in the workplace to prevent bullying and support bullied nurses.

CURRENT STATE OF WORKPLACE BULLYING LAW

- Bullying often involves abuse of power (ANA, 2015a). It comes as no surprise that the 2014 Workplace Bullying Institute's U.S. Workplace Bullying Survey found that most bullies are bosses. In nursing, this translates to managers, charge nurses, directors, and senior staff nurses (Healthy Workplace Bill [HWB], 2015). As a result, nurses may experience passive-aggressive, subtle uncivil, and humiliating conduct that is nearly impossible to prove.
- According to HWB (2015), 80% of bullying is legal. This speaks to the fact that most states have not enacted specific workplace bullying laws. Although there are laws that

protect against discrimination, nurses affected by abusive conduct have to fit as a protected class member to be protected under the law.

- Although there are specific laws against bullying, general anti-bullying laws focus on protecting children by preventing bullying in school districts (Duncan, 2011). Thus, these laws do not apply to nurses in the workplace setting.

Fast Facts in a Nutshell

The main problem with bullying in the workplace is that there is no statutory or case law action against workplace bullying, so employers are not inclined to have bullying preventive policies in place.

- Apparent bullying preventive policies derive from the lateral violence prevention mandates from accrediting bodies, such as The Joint Commission, and are not a deterrent to abusive conduct. These policies provide a mechanism only for internal reporting of lateral violence conduct with no real legal bite because there is no legislative requirement. Moreover, health care organizations are under pressure to develop and implement "No Tolerance" polices to satisfy Workplace Violence Prevention (WVP) state legislation. WVP laws are meant to prevent violence. Although some workplace bullying may rise to the level of violence, oftentimes it does not involve violence at all. In many cases, bullying conduct is neither discernable nor prevented under the WVP legislation. Therefore, although some internal policies may provide nurses with an internal process to deal with offensive conduct, they do not serve as the basis for a legal remedy.

LEGAL CLAIMS IN THE ABSENCE OF WORKPLACE BULLYING LAWS

Because there are no federal or state statutory laws that give rise to a legal claim of actions for workplace bullying, nurses who are the victims of bullying in their workplace must bring these legal actions under general workplace claims in tort, contract, or constitutional law.

A tort is a civil wrong against another person. A tort can be intentional, such as punching someone in the face, or unintentional, such as the tort of negligence. As a general matter, when nurses talk about a tort in health care, it refers to professional negligence as it relates to a deviation of a standard of care wherein the claimant has to prove that the nurse had a duty to act within the standard of care, the nurse breached that duty, or the nurse's conduct caused the injury and the claimant suffered damages.

Fast Facts in a Nutshell

Nurses who are the victims of bullying in the workplace must bring legal actions under general workplace claims in tort, contract, or constitutional law.

When bullying conduct in the workplace rises to the level of a tort, it can be of negligence but it is more likely intentional in nature. An intentional tort can be defined as a deliberate civil wrong by one person against another person. If the tort is intentional, the nurse can seek relief in the court against the perpetrator under civil theories of liability such as assault, battery, harassment, or defamation. In cases of tortious assault, the nurse must prove an overt act of hostility that puts the nurse in fear of harm. Civil battery requires proof of unconsented offensive touch. To prove harassment, the nurse must have been repeatedly subjected to the tortious conduct.

Raess v. Doescher (2008) may be considered the seminal case in terms of workplace bullying because of the expert's testimony about workplace bullying, although in reality the claimant sued for the tort of assault. The Indiana Supreme Court affirmed a jury award of $325,000 for assault of a perfusionist (heart–lung machine operator in open heart surgeries) who brought an action against a surgeon for an altercation in the hospital. The conduct alleged included coming at the plaintiff aggressively and rapidly with clenched fists, piercing eyes, beet-red face while screaming profanities at the plaintiff because of a report to the administration about his abuse of other perfusionists. The plaintiff feared he was going to be hit. The defendant stopped short of hitting him but threatened the plaintiff by stating "You're finished, you're history" (*Raess v. Doescher*, 2008).

Of note in this case is that in affirming the jury's award, the Court rejected the defendant's challenge to the plaintiff's expert testimony about workplace bullying. In the end, this case does not create a legal claim for workplace bullying. However, it may serve to caution employers to take bullying conduct more seriously and hopefully support an abuse-free culture (Yamada, 2005).

Another common claim for a workplace tort, which can be alleged by a nurse who is bullied in the workplace, is intentional infliction of emotional distress. A nurse who makes this claim must prove that the defendant committed an intentional act that is so "extreme and outrageous," causing severe emotional distress that no reasonable person should have to endure. Winning this claim is fact-dependent and relies heavily on a state's interpretation of this theory of liability.

In *Hollomon v. Keadle* (1996), for example, the Arkansas Supreme Court dismissed plaintiff's claim for intentional infliction of emotional distress, although her supervisor subjected her to repeated acts of bullying behaviors and her health was adversely affected, because she did not indicate to her supervisor that she was especially sensitive to such behaviors (326 Ark.

168. 931 S.W.2d 413 [Ark. 1991]). This holding is consistent with the results of a Workplace Bullying Institute study, which found that U.S. employers won 73% of the time in workplace bullying cases (Bible, 2012).

Nurses can also claim other tort theories of liability as redress for bullying conduct in the workplace (Bible, 2012). However, these claims are based largely on state law and thus turn on specific facts of the case. Some of these theories of liability are:

- **Tortious Interference With a Contract or Business Relationship**—Claimed when a nurse is forced to resign because of employer or coemployee tortious conduct and suffers damages because prospective employers will not hire him or her due to interference by offending employer.
- **Hostile Work Environment Harassment**—Claimed when a nurse is forced to endure harassment (sexual or otherwise) or is witness to the harassment of other nurses in the workplace and the organization fails to intervene.
- **Constructive Discharge**—Claimed when a nurse is forced to resign due to employer or coworker tortious conduct.
- **Defamation and Slander**—Claimed when a nurse is subjected to written or stated falsehoods from employer or coemployee and suffers damages to his or her professional reputation.
- **Respondeat Superior or Negligent Hiring/Supervision**—Wherein organizations can be held vicariously liable for the (negligent) acts of their employees.

Nurses may also draw upon some federal statutes for bullying conduct redress (Bible, 2012). Nurses who allege violations of statutory provisions under federal laws may have to meet "protected class" status (a person or class defined in the law). Moreover, they may have to exhaust their rights through the appropriate administrative agencies prior to filing a suit. Some of these statutes include:

- The Age Discrimination and Employment Act (ADEA), which prohibits discrimination based on age.
- Title VII of the Civil Rights Act of 1964, which prohibits discrimination based on race, color, religion, sex, or national origin.
- The Occupational Safety and Health Act (OSHA) of 1970 prohibits workplace bullying under the General Duty Clause (29 CFR 1910.5[a][1]). Nurses can report an employer to OSHA when job performance and safety have been adversely impacted by a coworker's bullying conduct causing injury. If the employer is found in violation of the Act, the bullied victim can file suit against all responsible parties including the employer.

Workers' compensation laws also provide a means for protection related to compensation and treatment for work-related injuries caused or exacerbated by workplace bullying conduct during the course of employment. Workers' compensation laws require employers to provide employees insurance for work-related injuries. However, these laws generally place restrictions on the employee's right to sue the health care entity. A nurse who has suffered primary injuries or exacerbation of injuries within the course of employment may qualify for workers' compensation benefits but may not be able to sue the employer for the bullying acts of employees. Yet, some states may allow for individual redress against the bully.

NURSING IMPLICATIONS FOR WORKPLACE BULLYING LEGISLATION

Although workplace bullying is not against the law in most states, 29 states and two U.S. territories have introduced versions of workplace anti-bullying bills (Health Workplace Bills [HWBs]). California, Tennessee, Utah, and North Dakota have enacted legislation that in effect outlaws workplace bullying.

According to a study of 612 staff nurses conducted by Spence Laschinger, Leitter, Day, and Gilin (2009), 67.5% reported being bullied by their supervisors and 77.6% by their coworkers. Nurses appear to be twice as likely to have experienced bullying compared to a Workplace Bullying Institute's study wherein 35% of U.S. non-health care workers reported workplace incivility (Workplace Bullying Institute, 2017).

The ANA's position statement on *Incivility, Bullying, and Workplace Violence* (2015b) provides a proper starting point for nurses who need guidance in terms of anti-bullying recommendations. The position statement includes information on:

- Continuing education in bullying prevention
- Reporting of bullying
- Working with the employer organization to develop policies and influence the culture
- Providing support to colleagues who are being bullied

The HWB legislation model was proposed by Professor David Yamada (2015) to prohibit abusive conduct in the workplace. This model for legislation provides guidance in terms of defining "abusive conduct" and determining the elements that would have to be met to find workplace conduct abusive (Melnick, 2014). For example, in HWB introduced in New York, "abusive work environment" is defined as "an employment condition where an employer or one or more of its employees, acting with intent to cause pain or distress *to an employee, subjects an employee to abusive conduct* that causes physical harm, psychological harm, or both" (Melnick, 2014). The American Bar Association (ABA) interprets the elements to meet this definition to be the following:

- Conduct that a reasonable person would find abusive
- More than one act of abusive conduct
- Increased penalties if the conduct is directed at someone with a disability

According to HWB (2015), the goal of HWB is to end abusive work environments by:

- Preventing bullying
- Providing self-help protections to encourage employers to prevent bullying employees to avail themselves of protective policies
- Providing relief to bully victims
- Allowing for monetary compensation
- Enforcing punishment for misconduct
- Defining "abusive conduct"
- Determining elements that identify an abusive work environment

Other countries are ahead of the United States in the fight against workplace bullying. Australia has enacted laws that criminalize workplace bullying (Epstein & Vogel, 2015), whereby a person who violates the law can be sentenced to prison. Five Canadian provinces have enacted or amended existing laws to make workplace bullying illegal, and in Europe, Sweden, England, and Ireland have enacted anti-bullying legislation (Epstein & Vogel, 2015).

Nurses must get involved in this movement. The Workplace Bullying Institute, a research, educational, and advocacy organization founded by renowned workplace bullying experts, Drs. Ruth and Gary Namie, is a great resource to learn about workplace bullying (Workplace Bullying Institute). Nurses should advocate in support of the HWB in their states because state laws can impose obligations on employers to develop preventive policies and work toward a common work culture free of bullying (HWB, 2015).

Nurses can join the campaign to eradicate workplace bullying by:

- Becoming educated about workplace bullying
- Reporting witnessed incidents of workplace bullying of others

- Reporting incidents of being bullied
- Developing and implementing preventive workplace policies
- Educating other nurses, nursing students, and the general public about workplace bullying
- Contacting local legislators to support introducing the HWB in their states
- Becoming a change agent of workplace culture

ASK A LAWYER

CASE STUDY 1

A nurse who worked on a maternity unit in a medical center for about 25 years has been the subject of repeated and continuous bullying from coworkers and supervisors for a 2-year period. One day she received a note from the unit secretary that stated: "Blond Fat Ass (Expletive) . . . Keep Eating, Looking at Cruises, and Singing Your Idol Songs. We Love It". Other nurses took part in this incident. The bullied nurse resigned while on workers' compensation.

What Were the Nurse's Legal Rights?

The nurse sued the hospital, nurse coworkers, and the secretary. Because the workers' compensation law of that state prohibited the hospital and nurse coworkers to be named, she could only allege intentional infliction of emotional distress against the secretary who left the unit shortly after the note was sent and had no other direct contact with her.

The Outcome

The U.S. District Court of Maine granted a motion to dismiss, holding that sending a note with abusive language with no further involvement does not rise to the level of "outrageous and extreme conduct" to support a claim of intentional infliction of emotional distress (*Pierre v. Eastern Maine Medical Center*, 2013).

CASE STUDY 2

A surgeon grabbed an operating room nurse by her shoulder, pulling her into the surgical site while screaming at her—"Can't you see where I'm working? I'm working in a hole. I need long instruments"—because he claimed she handed him the wrong instrument. He further berated her to others in the OR, calling her "incompetent."

What Were the Nurse's Legal Rights?

The nurse sued the surgeon, claiming intentional infliction of emotional distress, slander, and civil battery.

The Outcome

The trial court held for the defendant surgeon, dismissing the entire complaint. On appeal, the Ohio Court of Appeals reversed and remanded for trial the claim for slander and civil battery, finding that the surgeon intended the offensive contact and that his statements were sufficiently published. However, the Court affirmed the dismissal of the claim for intentional infliction of emotional distress (*Snyder v. Turk*, 1993).

References

Age Discrimination and Employment Act, 29 U.S.C. § 621 *et seq* (1967).

American Nurses Association. (2015a). *Code of ethics for nurses with interpretive statements*. Washington, DC: Author. Retrieved from http://nursingworld.org/DocumentVault/Ethics-1/Code-of-Ethics-for-Nurses.html

American Nurses Association. (2015b). *Incivility, bullying, and workplace violence*. Washington, DC: Author. Retrieved from http://www.nursingworld.org/MainMenuCategories/WorkplaceSafety/

Healthy-Nurse/bullyingworkplaceviolence/Incivility-Bullying-and-Workplace-Violence.html

Bible, J. D. (2012). The jerk at work: Workplace bullying and the law's inability to combat it. *Employee Relations Law Journal, 38*(1), 32–51.

Civil Rights Act of 1964, 42 U.S.C. § 2000e *et seq* (1964).

Duncan, S. H. (2011). Restorative justice and bullying: A missing solution in the antibullying laws. *New England Journal on Criminal and Civil Confinement, 37*(2), 267–298.

Epstein, D. E., & Vogel, A. J. (2015). The Healthy Workplace Act: Legislating "civility" in the workplace. Retrieved from http://news.acca.com/accnj/issues/2015-05-01/2.html

Healthy Workplace Bill. (2015). Retrieved from http://healthyworkplacebill.org

Hollomon v. Keadle, 326 Ark. 168, 931 S.W.2d 413 (1996)

Melnick, R. (2014). Understanding workplace-bullying legislation. Retrieved from http://apps.americanbar.org/litigation/committees/employment/articles/summer2014-0814-understanding-workplace-bullying-legislation.html

Pierre v. Eastern Maine Medical Center, No. 1: 12-cv-0265-NT (D. Me. Sept. 30, 2013).

Raess v. Doescher, 858 N.E.2d 790 (Ind. 2008). Retrieved from http://www.in.gov/judiciary/opinions/pdf/04080801bd.pdf

Snyder v. Turk, 62 N.E.2d 1053 (Ohio. Ct. App. 1993).

Spence Laschinger, H. K., Leitter, M., Day, A., & Gilin, D. (2009). Workplace empowerment, incivility, and burnout: Impact on staff nurse recruitment and retention outcomes. *Journal of Nursing Management, 17,* 302–311. doi:10.1111/j.1365-2834.2009.00999.x

Workplace Bullying Institute. (2017). Retrieved from http://www.workplacebullying.org

Yamada, D. C. (2005). Workplace bullying in healthcare III: A sampling of legal cases. Retrieved from https://newworkplace.wordpress.com/2009/12/22/workplace-bullying-in-healthcare-iii-a-sampling-of-legal-cases

Yamada, D. C. (2015). Workplace bullying and the law: U.S. legislative developments 2013-15. *Employee Rights and Employment Policy Journal, 19*(1), 49–59.

11

Bullying and the Student Nurse

What students learn and what they experience, either positive or negative, during their formation as a nurse will forever become part of their character. Horizontal violence is common among student nurses for many reasons and perpetuated because nurses see themselves as powerless. Unfortunately, much research on violence and bullying in nursing usually excludes student nurses in sample populations, and there have been few or no studies done on the correlation of horizontal violence and bullying and the effect on student nurses. Not only are student nurses victims of bullying, but they themselves become bullies as well. This impact must be addressed as well, because they are our future in the health care system, and the lives of patients depend on the student nurse becoming a just and moral citizen.

After reading this chapter, the reader will be able to:

- List 10 bullying behaviors toward nursing students
- Describe five physical effects of bullying on the student
- List how clinical instructors should support student nurses

(continued)

- List how preceptors should support student nurses
- Describe how schools of nursing should prepare students to deal with bullying

BULLYING *OF* THE STUDENT NURSE

Currently in the United States, the average age of a working nurse is older than 45. Therefore, it can be assumed that the student nurse of today will be part of the workforce in the future.

Fast Facts in a Nutshell

"Many student nurses . . . accept horizontal violence as a 'rite of passage,' only to mimic and repeat the behavior later in their careers" (Hinchberger, 2009, p. 43).

Nursing students compete for entrance to nursing school; this pits them against their peers. Then, once in nursing school, they are often met not with a warm welcome, but with an instructor who says, "Look on either side of you; that student won't be with you when you graduate." This introduces fear of failure and adds to an already stressful environment. The degradation of students continues throughout their clinical rotations and classroom attendance. At the end of their schooling, they then must compete for intern placements, academic honors, and job placement (not to mention NCLEX scores). This struggle does not create a colleague but rather a competitor against whom the student must win or face failure.

Nursing students suffer from lack of sleep, lack of a social outlet, intense worry, stress, and anxiety. Unless they have developed healthy coping mechanisms, this stress is turned outward onto fellow students, faculty, and family, resulting in negative comments and behavior and angry outbursts. Students may also face bullying from several different sources, including staff nurses, clinical and classroom instructors, patients, instructors, visitors, and fellow students.

BY THE NUMBERS

The bullying of nursing students, like that of their already graduated colleagues, exists universally.

- A 2002 New Zealand study noted that 170 nursing students had experienced "a distressing event" and one in three considered leaving nursing school. Fourteen considered leaving due to outright bullying (Clarke, Kane, Rajacich, & Lafreniere, 2012, p. 269).
- A 2007 study in Australia noted that 57% of nursing students had experienced or witnessed bullying (Clarke et al., 2012, p. 270).
- A 2006 study in the United Kingdom found that 53% of nursing students had experienced negative interactions during their clinical rotations (Clarke et al., 2012, p. 170).
- A 2004 study in Turkey found that 57.7% of nursing students had experienced verbal abuse and 69.5% had experienced academic abuse, and all thought of leaving the profession (Clarke et al., 2012, p. 269).
  - The term *academic abuse* is a term used to describe the bullying academia uses against students including negative remarks about the student becoming a nurse, clinical assignments meant to punish rather than for clinical education, assigning poor grades that were not earned or outright hostile treatment following academic achievement.
- According to the website www.stopbullyingnurses.com, 90% of nursing students reported being bullied by their instructors and staff nurses. In another study, 100% of

students responding have either experienced or observed violence in their clinical placements.

- One study of bachelor of science in nursing (BSN) nurses found that nearly 90% "noted difficulty confronting someone who was demonstrating horizontal/lateral violence. This lack of skill reflects the importance of conflict resolution training . . ." (Lachman, 2015, p. 39).

TYPES OF BULLYING EXPERIENCED BY STUDENT NURSES

Fast Facts in a Nutshell

The most common type of bullying against student nurses is verbal assault.

One study noted that clinical instructors were "identified as the greatest source of bullying behaviors in the practice setting" (Clarke et al., 2012, p. 272), followed by staff nurses, classmates, and patients. Other bullying behaviors experienced by students include the following:

- Being excluded or alienated
- Receiving *destructive* criticism from others (physicians, clinical instructors, professors, staff nurses, preceptors)
- Experiencing the resentment of staff nurses and/or fellow student nurses
- Being humiliated by a clinical instructor, preceptor, staff nurse, or physician in the presence of others
- Their work being undervalued by staff and clinical instructors
- Being subjected to negative remarks about them becoming a nurse (usually by staff nurses)
- Feeling that they are unfairly treated or treated differently than fellow students

- Staff nurses who are rude or who speak to them in a condescending manner
- Staff nurses who are sarcastic, patronizing, or who speak to them in a degrading manner
- Faculty, clinical instructors, and preceptors setting impossible expectations
- Being treated with hostility
- Made to feel like they are "in the way" and unwelcome on the unit
- Failure of basic courtesies such as ignoring an introduction or failure to make eye contact when being spoken to
- Refusing to answer questions when students are seeking help or guidance
- Failure of a staff nurse to follow up on clinical findings of patients when reported by students
- Repeating an action or care that students have already completed (e.g., vital signs, assessments)
- Being blamed for patient incidents that were, in reality, caused by the staff
- Being ignored by staff or the preceptor
- Lack of communication from staff nurses regarding patient care
- Feeling undue pressure to produce work
- Being lied about
- Being threatened with a poor evaluation by a clinical instructor
- Changing clinical expectations without informing students
- Classmates were noted as displaying the following bullying behavior: inappropriate jokes, spreading rumors, treating unfairly due to race, and teasing
- Patients and significant others bullying by verbal abuse, physical threats, and physical abuse
- Faculty who belittle or taunt students or who act cold and distant toward them

- Faculty being inflexible and rigid with rules in both class and clinical settings
- Faculty who are not available to students outside of class or who have office times that are not convenient to large numbers of students
- Faculty who are reluctant to answer students' questions or if the answer to a question is not known to seek out the answer
- Faculty who are unprepared for class or who verbalize their disinterest in the subject
- Faculty who attempt to "mentally sabotage" students by telling them how difficult an exam will be or how difficult it will be to pass the course
- Faculty who ignore disruptive students or who fail to discipline disruptive students
- Faculty not speaking clearly or not presenting information clearly

THE EFFECT ON THE STUDENT

All of bullying forces converge against the student, not allowing him or her to reach full potential. Bullying has a direct effect on the confidence level of the student and causes personal and professional outcomes similar to those of staff nurses, including the following:

- Decreased self-esteem
- Loss of autonomy
- Decreased self-worth
- Anger
- Fears
- Low morale
- Decreased productivity
- Frustration
- Increased errors
- Anxiety

- Stress
- Signs of burnout
- Apathy
- Passive anger
- Distancing themselves from friends, family, and patients
- Guilt
- Worry
- Fatigue
- Self-hatred
- Increase in absences and sickness from either physical or psychosomatic illness
- Sleep disturbances
- Symptoms similar to posttraumatic stress disorder (PTSD)

ADDRESSING THE SITUATION

It is the professional and ethical responsibility of faculty within schools of nursing and individual nurse educators to educate their students, beginning early in the process, to recognize signs of bullying from all persons with whom they currently interact or will interact in the future, including patients, staff, fellow students, instructors/professors, preceptors, and visitors, and to suggest strategies for a solution and to support changes in how bullying is addressed. Many colleges and universities do not act to remove a professor because he or she is tenured, so instead, the perpetrator may be moved to a different department or to another organization, still with easy access to students.

- Students should be educated (as all nurses should be) in what bullying and horizontal and lateral violence are and their impact on patient care—students could role-play different scenarios and educators should provide feedback regarding effective/ineffective communication.
  - Prepare students prior to entering the clinical area for bullying behaviors they may encounter and how to manage those behaviors.

    - Prior to graduation, again prepare students for behaviors they may encounter at a new job and how to manage those behaviors.
    - Allow students to freely express themselves about negative interactions they have encountered and how they dealt with the behavior—this sharing may assist a fellow student and could take place during post-conference time or in an open-classroom discussion.
    - Role-playing and conflict resolution should not be considered the cure for the bully or the victim. These strategies may actually encourage further bullying behavior if the school of nursing does not utilize other strategies to recognize and end the behavior.
- Nurse educators and staff development professionals should ensure that those who precept new nurses or students are educated in how to effectively precept. Do not pick an RN to be a preceptor because it is his or her turn, but rather because the RN wants to assist new nurses. Ensure that those who precept are properly compensated.
    - In one study, new nurses stated that they felt intimidated by their preceptors during orientation—orientation to a new unit or facility should be reviewed and modified to ensure that bullying behaviors are not evident and not passed onto new employees.
    - Preceptors often fail to effectively deal with students who exhibit bullying behaviors (poor attitude, improper communication style, lack of respect) because they have not been properly educated on how to precept. They lack the student/new nurse assessment skills and fall back on claiming that they do not want to upset the student instead of administering fair discipline.
    - Preceptors need to be given clear evaluation guidelines not only of the students' clinical skills but of their social skills as well.

  - Preceptors need to be considered part of the team (school faculty and clinical area preceptor) that ultimately decides if a student is prepared for a position in the health care field.
- Students should be taught whom they need to inform if bullying or violence occurs. The school and health care facility policies and procedures regarding bullying reporting must be reviewed with the student. This includes witnesses to bullying.
- Students, in turn, must feel safe in reporting to their instructor, faculty, preceptor, and, later on, to a unit manager. They must feel that their complaints are taken seriously and will be acted upon and are held in confidence.
- All educators including preceptors should be knowledgeable in the methods to resist bullying and horizontal violence as well as to identify it.
- It may be helpful to assign a mentor to a student who is not on the clinical unit. That way, the student has a "safe" person to whom he or she can communicate any issues.
- Educators, in every venue, classroom, clinical area, and so forth, must model behavior that includes effective methods for reducing hostility.
- Educators must not be seen as tolerating abuse, bullying, or violence—they should model that nothing but respect will be tolerated from any health care professional, student, patient, or visitor.
- Student nurses need to be taught that violence, bullying, and verbal abuse are *not* part of nursing, and enduring them are *not* a rite of passage!
- Student nurses must recognize that we as nurses do not provide our caring and compassion just for our patients, but for all whom we meet and with whom we work.
- *All* nurses should model professional behavior! What is seen by students is imitated by them. If students experience

bullying and the bullying is condoned, they will become bullies and the cycle continues.

- Clinical instructors should be knowledgeable in not only clinical skills but also in how to effectively communicate and interact with students and fellow staff.
    - Clinical instructors should receive an in-depth orientation and should have faculty members as a source of support.
    - Clinical instructors should be educated in how to provide constructive criticism, ongoing feedback, and effective evaluations.
    - Clinical instructors should be able to build the strengths of the student, not knock them down. Instructors should support students' efforts and act as their advocates.
- "Student nurses . . . should be taught that if the behavior is offensive and undermines them on their job in any way, it is probably horizontal violence and should be reported" (Hinchberger, 2009, p. 43).
- All nursing schools and universities have a responsibility to define bullying, and to design and implement anti-bullying policies and procedures.
- Students should be provided with information of outside or university support of a victim of bullying. This can include the health care facility where the bullying took place.
- Nursing faculty must become the gatekeepers, enforcing zero tolerance for bullying at anyone's hands (fellow faculty, clinical instructors, staff nurses, patients, family members, physicians, and classmates).
- Students should be made aware of the psychological effects of bullying and also coping mechanisms to deal with the stress.

Further exploration of these issues appears in Chapter 12, which presents case studies relating to bullying of the student nurse.

References

Clarke, C. M., Kane, D. J., Rajacich, D. L., & Lafreniere, K. D. (2012). Bullying in undergraduate clinical nursing education. *Journal of Nursing Education*, *51*(5), 269–276.

Hinchberger, P. A. (2009). Violence against female student nurses in the workplace. *Nursing Forum*, *44*(1), 38–46.

Lachman, V. D. (2015). Ethical issues in the disruptive behaviors of incivility, bullying, and horizontal/lateral violence. *Urology Nurse*, *35*(1), 39–42.

12

Case Studies: Bullying and the Student Nurse

The previous chapter described the bullying experienced by student nurses. This chapter explores three case studies illustrating such bullying, identifying the bullying behavior demonstrated along with the probable cause, victim intervention, potential witness interventions, and critical thinking moments.

After reading this chapter, the reader will be able to:

- List five bullying behaviors demonstrated against student nurses
- Describe how to assist the student nurse who is being bullied
- Describe the probable causes of student nurses being bullied
- List three witness interventions for the student nurse who is being bullied
- List what actions the student nurses can take after being bullied
- Identify the critical thinking moments in a bullying incident

CASE STUDY 1

Susan is a first-year nursing student. Today, she will be administering an insulin injection for the first time. As she stands with her clinical instructor by the medication cart, she carefully recites the medication side effects and other data she had memorized the evening before. The clinical instructor watches as Susan draws up the insulin, checks the amount against the physician's order, and double-checks the vial. The instructor walks with Susan into the patient room and watches as she approaches her patient and wipes the injection site on the patient's arm with alcohol. Just as Susan is about to inject the insulin, the instructor yells at her to stop and leave the room immediately. As they walk into the hall and in front of fellow students, staff, patients, and visitors, the instructor begins to berate Susan for not identifying the patient. The browbeating continues well into post-conference as the instructor makes an example of her to the other students as to what not to do when administering medication. Finally, Susan is told in front of her fellow students to expect a bad evaluation that will affect her final grade.

Bullying Behavior Demonstrated

- Being excluded or alienated
- Receiving *destructive* criticism from others (physicians, clinical instructors, professors, staff nurses, preceptors)
- Being humiliated by a clinical instructor, preceptor, staff nurse, or physician in the presence of others
- Being treated with hostility
- Being threatened with a poor evaluation by a clinical instructor
- Experiencing faculty who belittle or taunt students or who act cold and distant toward them

Probable Cause

- Being a student nurse (because such nurses are new, lack confidence, and are powerless)

- The actions of the student not matching the "ideals" of a preceptor, clinical instructor, or faculty member
- Faculty, preceptorship, clinical instructor focusing on the evaluation or end result, rather than learning

Victim Intervention

- See Box 12.1.
- Try not to be afraid. Fear will prevent you from taking action against the behavior.
- Be aware that if you speak up and attempt to defend yourself, it may encourage the bully to continue the behavior.
- When documenting bullying, the fact that patient care is being impacted will be important to management.

Witness Intervention

- See Box 12.2.
- Let the bully know that what he or she has done has been witnessed.
- Let the bully know that his or her actions are not consistent with the policies of the school.

Critical Thinking Moment

- As a staff nurse, have you ever witnessed bullying of a student by a clinical instructor? If so, how did you handle the situation? Was it effective?
- In the future, if you witness a student being bullied, how will you handle the situation?
- Have you ever addressed the bully or reported the incident? If not, why not?
- If you are a clinical instructor or preceptor, how do you approach a student who has made an error?

CASE STUDY 2

Samantha was a first-term diploma student. She was so proud and thrilled to be in nursing school and had just started working with patients. She loved caring for them and speaking with them. She felt that she had found her niche. Not many people knew that when Samantha was nervous, she stuttered and had difficulty expressing herself. She hoped that this would not prevent her from caring for her patients. One day during preconference, the professor who was the clinical instructor went around the group of students asking the usual questions about the patients they would care for during the clinical day. The students responded, telling the instructor about past medical histories, current medications, and care to be administered. The instructor began asking Samantha the same questions; however, Samantha had forgotten a piece of her research. She was unable to answer the instructor's questions. The instructor began voicing the questions in rapid-fire succession, and Samantha became so nervous and stressed that she was unable to speak and began to stutter when she tried. To the other students, it was as if the instructor was a shark who sensed blood in the water. Samantha began to cry as the questions became more and more demanding on points she could not answer. She was so stressed that her hands and voice were shaking. In triumph, it seemed to the other students, the instructor finally stopped and announced to the students and Samantha that if Samantha could not speak without stuttering, she could not care for patients. Samantha was so humiliated that she left the school after that day and never became a nurse.

Bullying Behavior Demonstrated

- Humiliating and belittling students
- Not being emotionally supportive

Probable Cause

- Being a student nurse (because such nurses are new, lack confidence, and are powerless)
- The actions of the student not matching the "ideals" of a preceptor, clinical instructor, or faculty member

Victim Intervention

- See Box 12.1.
- Be aware that if you speak up and attempt to defend yourself, it may encourage the bully to continue the behavior.
- When documenting bullying, the fact that patient care is being impacted will be important to management.

Witness Intervention

- See Box 12.2.
- Let the bully know that what he or she has done has been witnessed.
- Let the bully know that his or her actions are not consistent with the policies of the school.

Critical Thinking Moment

- As an educator, have you ever witnessed bullying of a student by another educator? If so, how did you handle the situation? Was it effective?
- In the future, if you witness a student being bullied, how will you handle the situation?
- Have you ever addressed the bully or reported the incident? If not, why not?
- If you are a clinical instructor or faculty, how do you approach a student who has made an error?

CASE STUDY 3

Elizabeth was a second-year diploma student. She had consistently received straight As in her academic work and outstanding clinical grades. She was voted president of her class and she thoroughly enjoyed nursing school because she was learning to be what she had always wanted to be.

Elizabeth was entering the cardiac clinical rotation. It was the rotation that all of the students dreaded, not because of the course content, but because of one specific nursing professor. Ms. Hart had a reputation of selecting one nursing student and "riding him or her" until he or she either failed out of the clinical rotation and had to repeat it or failed out of school altogether. It was not known why she did this; it was just accepted behavior and what had always been.

Unfortunately for Elizabeth, it was her turn to be the student chosen by Ms. Hart. The rotation started out as they all did. Elizabeth continued to receive good grades and tried to be on what she hoped was perceived as her best behavior. She worked long hours completing her preclinical research and gave all the required information when questioned in pre-conference. Then, one day, it all began to fall to pieces. She was assigned a patient who had recently had the left leg amputated. The patient weighed more than 300 lbs, but had orders to get out of bed to a geri-chair. After assisting the patient in completing their AM care, Elizabeth asked fellow students and staff to assist her in moving the patient. Ms. Hart gave Elizabeth an "unsatisfactory" grade for the day because she had asked for assistance. During another clinical day, Elizabeth was assigned a patient who was actively dying. At 19 years of age, Elizabeth had never been in this situation before and had attended only one funeral in her lifetime. She was emotionally unprepared for the challenge of caring for a dying person. She approached Ms. Hart about the appropriate things that should be done to care for the patient. At one point, Elizabeth started to cry, but was able to control her emotions and complete her care of the patient and the patient's family. She received an unsatisfactory grade for the day because Ms. Hart stated she needed emotional help to deal with her assignment. Elizabeth was distraught. If she received three unsatisfactory grades in clinical, she would be excused from the program. On the last day of clinical, Elizabeth was instructing a diabetic patient in how to inject insulin. She could see Ms. Hart pacing outside the patient's room. Elizabeth tried to ignore the pacing outside of the room and concentrate on the patient and her teaching. At the end of the clinical day, Ms. Hart approached Elizabeth and asked her why she was ignoring her. Elizabeth stated that she was attempting to instruct her patient. Ms. Hart stomped off, clearly angry with Elizabeth.

Elizabeth confided to her mother what had happened during her clinical rotation and stated that she no longer wanted to be a nurse, saying that there was something obviously wrong with how she cared for patients despite having done so well in the past. Her mother was Elizabeth's support system and told her that they would both go to speak to the dean of the school but that Elizabeth should speak to Ms. Hart. Elizabeth attempted to speak to Ms. Hart, but the conversation ended when she told Elizabeth she would never be a nurse because she could not handle taking care of patients. Elizabeth made an appointment with the dean and together with her mother told the dean what had happened and about the behavior of the professor. Because of her academic grades, Elizabeth did not fail out of clinical. She continued on to the next rotation where she received no more than satisfactory grades no matter how hard she tried. She was told at the end of clinical by the professor who was her instructor, Ms. Smith, that no other instructors wanted her in their rotation because they did not want to go against Ms. Hart. Ms. Smith told Elizabeth that the reason she had not received any grades higher than satisfactory was because as she stated, "no one would believe me." Elizabeth left the diploma school after this last rotation and was accepted at a nearby associate's degree program, weary and still questioning whether nursing was her correct path. At the end of the year, however, she graduated cum laude and went on to a very successful nursing career.

Bullying Behavior Demonstrated

- Receiving *destructive* criticism from others (physicians, clinical instructors, professors, staff nurses, preceptors)
- Being humiliated by a clinical instructor, preceptor, staff nurse, or physician in the presence of others
- Being subjected to negative remarks about becoming a nurse (usually by staff nurses)
- Feeling that they are unfairly treated or treated differently than fellow students
- Encountering staff nurses who are sarcastic, patronizing, or who speak to them in a degrading manner
- Experiencing faculty, clinical instructors, and preceptors setting impossible expectations
- Being treated with hostility
- Missing basic courtesies, such as ignoring an introduction or failure to make eye contact when being spoken to
- Being lied about
- Being threatened with a poor evaluation by a clinical instructor
- Experiencing faculty who belittle or taunt students or who act cold and distant toward them
- Experiencing faculty who are inflexible and rigid with rules in both class and clinical settings
- Experiencing faculty who attempt to "mentally sabotage" students by telling them how difficult an exam will be or how difficult it will be to pass the course

Probable Cause

- Being a student nurse (because such nurses are new, lack confidence, and feel powerless)
- The actions of the student not matching the "ideals" of a preceptor, clinical instructor, or faculty

Victim Intervention

- See Box 12.1.
- Be sure to have a support group of your peers or a trusted person to whom you can speak.

BOX 12.1 VICTIM INTERVENTIONS TO RESIST BULLYING OF THE STUDENT NURSE

- Don't ignore or excuse the behavior.
- Set limits on what you will tolerate from the bully.
- Be aware of school policies and procedures in dealing with hostile behavior and bullying, and to whom they should be reported.
- Try not to be afraid. Fear will prevent you from taking action against the behavior.
- Document the date, time, location, and those involved. Give specific details of what occurred including how you attempted to stop the behavior.
- Follow school policies on reporting the bullying episode.
- Note and document if the instructor bullying you also bullies other students. Be sure that all are documenting as well. More proof of bullying by multiple students will have more of an impact.
- Be aware of your own behaviors.
- Take care of you! Work stress reduction into your daily schedule.
- Be sure to have a support group of your peers or a trusted person to whom you can speak.
- Do not take matters into your own hands and retaliate against the perpetrator.
- Seek professional counseling if needed.

Witness Intervention

- See Box 12.2.

Critical Thinking Moment

- As an educator, have you ever witnessed bullying of a student by another educator? If so, how did you handle the situation? Was it effective?
- In the future, if you witness a student being bullied, how will you handle the situation?
- Have you ever addressed the bully or reported the incident? If not, why not?
- As a clinical instructor or preceptor, how do you approach a student who is emotionally upset due to a patient condition?
- As a clinical instructor or preceptor, do you use another student's mistake as an example to other students? If so, why? Should this practice be continued?

BOX 12.2 WITNESS INTERVENTIONS TO RESIST BULLYING OF THE STUDENT NURSE

- Take the complaint of bullying and incivility seriously.
- Suggest to the victim that there is a support system available. If the witness is not readily aware of the support system, support the victim in finding assistance.
- Be aware of unit/facility anti-bullying policies and procedures and inform the victim.
- Support the target of bullying in efforts to stand up to the abuse.
- Encourage the victim to report episodes of bullying to the school.

(continued)

- Allow the process of reporting to occur and support the victim during the process.
- Suggest counseling for the victim if he or she expresses a need for it because of emotional trauma that may have occurred.

13

Bullying and the Novice Nurse

As is widely known, a nurse's first position in the health care system forms the basis for how he or she regards the profession as a whole, now and in the future. New nurses enter the profession full of promise and excitement. They look forward to fulfilling lifelong goals of caring for patients and "making a difference in the world." They are often met, however, with behavior from more experienced nurses that causes them psychological distress and, more often than not, causes them to leave the profession.

After reading this chapter, the reader will be able to:

- Describe the role of the preceptor in preventing bullying of the novice nurse
- Describe how the preceptor can assist in decreasing bullying on the unit
- Describe the effects of bullying on the novice nurse
- Describe how to support the novice nurse who has been bullied
- Explain why the novice nurse may be reluctant to report being bullied

THE NOVICE NURSE

Very few studies have been conducted on the effects of bullying and the novice nurse. One study conducted by Griffin (2004) was completed at a large metropolitan hospital in the United States. Upon being hired, 26 newly graduated nurses were taught cognitive rehearsal techniques in order to deal with bullying. Cognitive rehearsal is a technique used in therapy between a therapist and a patient. The patient is able to rehearse how she or he would deal with a stressful situation with specific techniques while in the safety of a controlled environment. It is hoped that this better equips the patient to deal with a real-life situation. The goal of the program with the new nurses was to assist them in dealing with bullying and to prevent it from interfering with unit socialization and their future learning.

The patients, or the nurses in this case, were first taught about bullying and lateral violence in nursing. They were then given specific written cues on cards that contained appropriate verbal responses to the most common forms of bullying. A year later, it was found that the retention rate among the nurses was 91%, much higher than had been previously reported by the hospital. The nurses verbalized that they felt "empowered to confront the perpetrator of the abusive behaviors" (Chipps & McRury, 2012, p. 95). Another study in 2002 developed educational workshops aimed at nurse managers and supervisors in a facility with a known bullying concern. After the workshops, the retention rate increased (Chipps & McRury, 2012, p. 95).

Fast Facts in a Nutshell

Of all the levels of nursing, the one most vulnerable to bullying is the new graduate or novice nurse.

NOVICE NURSE BULLYING—THE STATISTICS

- According to Berry, Gillespie, Fisher, Gormley, and Haynes (2012), 73% of new nurses felt that they had been bullied within the past month
- According to Berry et al. (2012), 58% felt they were a direct target of a bully or bullies
- After 6 months of employment, 60% of new RNs in the United States quit their job due to some form of bullying (Flateau-Lux & Gravel, 2014, p. 227)

Fast Facts in a Nutshell

Bullying during the first months of new nurses' careers influences their decision to leave their place of employment—or the career of nursing altogether—more than any other factor.

Novice nurses are caught in a very difficult position. They are new employees, often young and inexperienced in social situations, and they are inexperienced in the profession. They are powerless and have not been taught to deal with and respond to bullying. If they speak up, they feel they will lose their jobs. The level of stress experienced by novice nurses who are being bullied

- Leads to not being able to correctly learn to care for their patients
- Causes an inability to concentrate and learn in the stressful, hostile environment
- Causes comprised patient care

THE ROLE OF THE PRECEPTOR

The book *Fast Facts for the Nurse Preceptor: Keys to Providing a Successful Preceptorship in a Nutshell* (Ciocco, 2015, pp. 104–108) emphasizes the importance of the preceptor in the formation of a registered professional nurse. The following passage is from that book:

> The preceptor must at all times provide guidance and support and be a model of professional nursing behavior. The preceptor must be aware of facility policies dealing with unprofessional conduct and know whom to contact if their preceptee becomes a victim of workplace bullying. Also, the preceptee:
>
> - Should not blame himself or herself for the behavior and actions of the bully. The preceptee should remember that bullies choose targets whom they find threatening, and a threat can be anything from how the preceptee looks to a perceived threat to job security.
> - Should be encouraged to objectively document the occurrence of bullying, including who, what, when, where, and how. Document conversations that took place, including word-for-word quotes.
> - Should not confuse the verbal abuse that the bully uses with "constructive criticism." The preceptee should instead focus on his or her accomplishments and maintain self-confidence.
> - Should not respond in kind to the bully (through rude or belittling behavior), but rather continue to work to the best of his or her ability.
> - Should be aware of the chain of command on the unit and within the facility when reporting bullying. The preceptee should be encouraged to report the incivility immediately to a unit manager, and should be aware of whom to report to if the unit manager does not act or if the unit manager is the bully.
> - Should be aware of all facility policies regarding workplace professional behavior and conduct.

- Should seek out support from a mentor or trusted friend. The preceptee can also research how to deal with a bully at www.workplacebullying.org

As a mentor and preceptor, be open to complaints of intimidation, humiliation, belittlement, or social isolation voiced to you by the preceptee. Assure the preceptee that the complaint will be handled without fear of reprisal. The preceptee should be free to verbalize issues that ultimately affect patient care. Assure the preceptee that you will work to find solutions and will bring the complaint to a higher authority if necessary. Other actions to take include the following:

- If the facility does not have a "zero-tolerance policy" when it comes to bullying nor policies and procedures to support zero-tolerance, then work to change that.
- Encourage a "clique-less" unit. As previously noted, cliques can have a negative impact on staff retention (especially as this relates to newly employed nurses).
- Support the person who was bullied in his or her efforts to stand up to the abuse. Many victims of bullying do not wish to openly confront a bully because they are uncomfortable with confrontation or afraid of retaliation. Counsel the preceptee that he or she may respond in a professional manner.
- Encourage the new nurse to report episodes of bullying to human resources or, in the case of the nursing student, per school policy, as appropriate.
- Allow the process of reporting to occur, including the processes for superiors to deal with the unprofessional behavior, and support the preceptee during the process.
- Suggest counseling for the victim if he or she expresses a need for it because of emotional trauma that may have occurred.

Further exploration of these issues appears in Chapter 14, which presents case studies relating to bullying of the novice nurse.

References

Berry, P., Gillespie, G., Fisher, B., Gormley, D., & Haynes, J. (2016) Psychological distress and workplace bullying among registered nurses. *OJIN: The Online Journal of Issues in Nursing, 21*(3), 8. doi: 10.3912/OJIN.Vol21No03PPT41

Chipps, E. M., & McRury, M. (2012). The development of an educational intervention to address workplace bullying. *Journal for Nurses in Staff Development, 28*(3), 94–98.

Ciocco, M. (2015). *Fast facts for the nurse preceptor: Keys to providing a successful preceptorship in a nutshell.* New York, NY: Springer Publishing.

Flateau-Lux, L. R., & Gravel, G. (2014). Put a stop to bullying new nurses. *Home Healthcare Nurse, 32*(4), 225–229.

Griffin, M. (2004). Teaching cognitive rehearsal as a shield for lateral violence: An intervention for newly licensed nurses. *The Journal of Continuing Education in Nursing, 35*(6), 257–263.

14

Case Studies: Bullying and the Novice Nurse

Although bullying of the novice nurse is similar to that of a student nurse, new nurses may not have a support system. They are alone in a new job with very little support from a preceptor or the staff.

After reading this chapter, the reader will be able to:

- List five bullying behaviors experienced by the novice nurse
- List the probable causes of bullying behavior against the novice nurse
- List five victim interventions for a novice nurse who is being bullied
- List five witness interventions for a novice nurse who is being bullied
- Explain why bullying of the novice nurse is similar to that of the student nurse
- Identify the critical thinking moments in a bullying incident

CASE STUDY 1

In this scenario, a recent graduate experiences bullying in her new job.

Angela just recently graduated from an associate degree program. At 23 years of age, she was one of the youngest students to graduate in her class and she was so proud to finally reach her goal of being a nurse! She was just hired to work 7 to 3 on a 36-bed medical–surgical unit. Because the unit manager was on vacation, she was interviewed and hired by the shift supervisor. She attended orientation as assigned and then began work on the unit.

On her first day, she was assigned a preceptor, Marybeth. Angela was told by a fellow new nurse that "Marybeth is the best preceptor; she is so smart and so nice!" She was introduced to the staff, many of whom seemed reluctant to greet her or get to know her. The unit manager, Rebecca, returned from vacation and Angela attempted to greet her with a friendly exchange, which Rebecca ignored. Instead, Rebecca looked Angela up and down and said, "Oh, look what happens when I leave the unit? What a surprise! I guess you're working here? I don't even know you and I'm not sure I want you!"

Angela was crushed. She tried to be positive, however, and continue her care, but she began to notice that every time she entered the nurses' station, all discussions seemed to stop and the nurses looked away. She would be left on the unit, whereas the other nurses went on their lunch break. If she asked Marybeth, her preceptor, for help on a procedure that Angela had never completed, she was met with eye-rolling and sighing. One time Marybeth asked Angela if she knew anything at all because a new bachelor of science in nursing (BSN) was also new to the unit and Marybeth stated "she was having no problems." She even heard Marybeth mocking her and laughing about a whispered joke about her one day in front of the other nurses. The charge nurse told Angela she was "too gung ho." She was given assignments that were difficult to complete, but she had no choice—she had to care for her patients. She would try to find someone to help transfer or reposition a patient and find the entire staff, including her preceptor, sitting at the nurses' station talking and laughing. She felt she was alone and had no one to go to for help or in whom to confide.

She decided she would have to help herself and researched any skill to be provided rather than to ask for assistance because she knew she would not get any. She heard from fellow graduate nurses that they were experiencing similar actions on their units. "Was this why I went into nursing?," she asked herself.

Bullying Behavior Demonstrated

- Being excluded or alienated
- Receiving destructive criticism from others (physicians, clinical instructors, professors, staff nurses, preceptors) in the presence of others
- Being subjected to negative remarks about becoming a nurse (usually by staff nurses)
- Feeling unfairly treated or treated differently than fellow nurses
- Encountering staff nurses who are rude or who speak to them in a condescending manner
- Being made to feel like they are "in the way" and unwelcome on the unit
- Missing basic courtesies, such as ignoring an introduction or failure to make eye contact when being spoken to
- Refusing to answer questions when students are seeking help or guidance
- Being ignored by staff or the preceptor
- Finding lack of communication from staff nurses regarding patient care

Probable Cause

- A form of control

- Just being a novice nurse (because such nurses are new, lack confidence, and are powerless)
- Being perceived as a threat to the status quo

Victim Intervention

- See Box 14.1.

Witness Intervention

- See Box 14.2.

Critical Thinking Moment

- Have you witnessed a staff nurse bullying a new nurse? How do you handle the situation?
- Have you ever addressed the bully or reported the incident? If not, why not?
- As a preceptor, how do you approach a new nurse who has made an error?
- As a preceptor or staff nurse, how do you answer a new nurse who asks for assistance?
- As a staff nurse, are you welcoming to a new nurse? If not, why not?
- As a staff nurse, how do you approach a new nurse who has made an error?
- As a preceptor, how do you address a fellow nurse who has bullied a new staff member?

CASE STUDY 2

In this scenario, an experienced nurse, new to a unit, takes on the role of the novice nurse and experiences the same bullying as her less-experienced counterpart.

Sara had graduated with her master of science in nursing (MSN) several years ago. She currently works as a clinical instructor at an associate's degree program, but wanted to work per diem to maintain her skills. She was eagerly hired by Julia, the nurse manager of a 40-bed unit within a large metropolitan hospital. Before she even began her work, she was introduced by Julia to the staff as a "watchdog," which made Sara cringe. The unit manager added, "She has an MSN, so she could teach you all a few things." The nursing staff just stared at Sara.

Sara began work after facility orientation on the 7 a.m. to 7 p.m. shift. On the first day, she was assigned a preceptor and 10 patients. Sara was told by the preceptor that because she was an experienced nurse, she could handle it. Sara started rounds and noted that of the 10 patients, 6 of them had IVs and they were all in various stages of running dry. One of her patients was actively dying. Rounding out the patient load were the usual types of medical–surgical patients, all requiring a.m. care and medications.

After rounds, Sara obtained report but it was rushed and did not have much detail. When Sara asked for further information, the nurse giving her the report just rolled her eyes and kept talking. During the morning, when it was evident that Sara was not going to receive any help with patient care, she was told by the charge nurse that the hospital was undergoing a transition and phasing out LPNs and the respiratory therapy department and eliminating nurse's aides. The RNs were expected to provide all bedside care, respiratory therapy, and conduct bedside tests, such as EKGs and drawing of blood for lab work. Sara had never learned how to administer respiratory meds nor had she ever done an EKG. Her preceptor told her to "just follow the directions" on the machine and to read up about respiratory therapy medications before administering them.

Sara was rushing around trying to complete all of her a.m. care alone when she was told she had an additional patient. This patient was not on her list in the morning, but had since been added after the shift was well underway. The patient had a history of AIDS, but was in isolation for another type of infection, putting Sara even further behind. Sara was becoming overwhelmed and angry. She was unable to keep up; no one was helping her. It was as if they were watching her struggle and taking great joy in it.

Sara had reviewed the medications to be given after receiving report, but now she was behind in their administration. A pharmacy tech showed up on the unit with medications and asked Sara to sign for narcotics. Sara noticed that the count was inaccurate and reported it to the charge nurse who told her, "Just sign for them, it'll be okay." Sara refused, which made the charge nurse angry. The patient who was dying was alone, and Sara felt awful that she could not be with him, but she was rushing to get a.m. care completed before it became any later in the afternoon.

When she finally caught up, she discovered the staff had gone to lunch, including her preceptor, without asking her if she needed help or if she wanted a break. Seven p.m. could not come soon enough, but she kept going, attempting to care for her patient load despite missing equipment and medications that the pharmacy never delivered. When the shift was over, she left 3 hours late. She told her husband she would never go back to work on that unit.

Bullying Behavior Demonstrated

- Being excluded or alienated
- Being ignored by staff or the preceptor
- Feeling the resentment of staff nurses
- Feeling unfairly treated or treated differently than fellow nurses
- Given patient care responsibilities with no mentor/preceptor or other more experienced nurse supervision
- Having patient care information withheld by another nurse
- Preceptors or other staff setting impossible expectations

- Given an unmanageable work load or patient care that is not familiar
- Missing basic courtesies such as ignoring an introduction or failure to make eye contact when being spoken to
- Refusing to answer questions when students are seeking help or guidance
- Having little, no, or poor orientation
- Not being given support by the preceptor (emotionally, especially when experiencing reality shock)
- Not being given report by the staff so that correct care could take place
- Unit orientation that was too brief or nonexistent or poorly provided

Probable Cause

- A form of control
- Jealousy regarding the educational level of the new nurse in contrast to the staff nurses
- Undue favoritism placed on the new nurse by the unit manager and resentment of the new nurse's role
- Hostility toward those who are perceived as being intelligent, competent, and accomplished
- Being a seasoned nurse, but new to a unit or facility
- A lack of resources or equipment to properly and safely care for patients
- Working short-staffed

Victim Intervention

- See Box 14.1.

Witness Intervention

- See Box 14.2.

Critical Thinking Moment

- Have you witnessed a staff nurse bullying an employee? How did you handle the situation?
- Have you ever addressed a bully or reported the incident? If not, why not?
- How do you answer and help a new nurse who needs assistance?
- Have you ever asked a new nurse to go against unit/facility policy "just to see what will happen?"
- As a staff nurse, are you welcoming to a new nurse? If not, why not?
- As a preceptor, how do you address a fellow nurse who has bullied a new staff member?

BOX 14.1 VICTIM INTERVENTIONS TO RESIST BULLYING OF THE NOVICE NURSE

- One should not blame himself or herself for the behavior of others.
- Document the occurrence of bullying, including who, what, when, where, and how.
- Do not confuse verbal abuse with "constructive criticism."
- Be aware of the chain of command on the unit and within the facility when reporting bullying.
- Be aware of whom to report to if the unit manager does not act or if the unit manager is the bully.
- Be aware of all facility policies regarding workplace professional behavior and conduct.
- Seek out support from a mentor or trusted friend.

BOX 14.2 WITNESS INTERVENTIONS TO RESIST BULLYING OF THE NOVICE NURSE

- Take the complaint of bullying and incivility seriously.
- Be aware of unit/facility anti-bullying policies and procedures and inform the victim.
- Support the target of bullying in efforts to stand up to the abuse.
- Counsel the victim that he or she may respond in a professional manner.
- Encourage the victim to report episodes of bullying to human resources.
- Allow the process of reporting to occur and support the preceptee during the process.
- Suggest counseling for the victim if he or she expresses a need for it because of emotional trauma that may have occurred.

15

Bullying in Nursing Education

Academia should be the considered the foundation of the movement to end bullying, but it is often where bullying in nursing begins.

After reading this chapter, the reader will be able to:

- List five root causes of bullying in nursing education
- List 10 bullying behaviors found in nursing education
- List 10 bullying behaviors demonstrated by the student nurse
- List five ways bullying nursing education can be decreased
- Describe how nursing staff may be stressed by the presence of nurse educators on the nursing unit

Fast Facts in a Nutshell

The bullying behavior demonstrated and experienced by nurses in the workplace has its roots in the nursing school, where some nurse educators often sit in judgment of students and fellow educators, fueling the need to assert superiority.

ROOT CAUSES

Academia, like all areas of nursing, has long-standing traditions and expectations. Bullying among faculty is also viewed as a rite of passage and considered the "norm." One study conducted in 2013 found that bullying in academia is worldwide but is particularly highest in Anglo-American universities (Birks, 2014, p. 1685). This would suggest that culture plays a large part in the existence of bullying at a university so it is also surmised that neoliberalism (defined as an outgrowth of liberalism that is not as pro-union or suspicious of militarism as traditional liberalism) is the reason it has such a high prevalence in Anglo-American universities. In other words, a university no longer exists to educate, but rather to make money and students are seen as "clients" and "autonomy of academics is reduced" (Birks, 2014, p. 1685).

Other causes of bullying in schools of nursing are the following:

- There is pressure to change how education is delivered, increase student numbers, decrease attrition, and increase NCLEX passage rates to maintain the academic standing.
- Faculty are often asked to "do more with less and do it differently," increasing their stress.
- Historically, faculty are unwilling to deal with rapid change in how education is delivered.
- Bullying usually occurs in institutions that are struggling to survive. So, a dean may be bullied by a school president, and the dean may then bully and harass subordinate staff and faculty members.
- Pressure is placed on faculty to retain students, irrespective of their behavior or lack of academic integrity.
- Faculty and staff may fear being sued by the students.
- Faculty lack support from school administration to discipline students who bully.
- Disciplining a student nurse if he or she is seen to be uncaring and not consistent with the ideals of the profession of nursing.

Other causes include:

- Workload inequality
- Lack of time to maintain clinical competence
- Inability to advance
- Lack of administrative support
- High faculty turnover or movement of staff from full time to part time due to financial issues of the school
- Poor coping skills
- Student behavior or clinical issues

Like other forms of bullying in nursing, bullying in academia is often not reported. It is surmised that anti-bullying policies are not in effect for academia at this time, although teaching nursing students how to recognize and combat bullying is becoming more common.

BULLYING BEHAVIORS SPECIFIC TO ACADEMIA

There are several types of bullying among faculty. There is vertical violence or bullying from dean to faculty and faculty to dean or higher, and horizontal bullying among faculty members. The actions seen include the overt aggression previously spoken about in previous chapters. However, there are also actions seen in vertical bullying that are very often more difficult to distinguish. Bullying behaviors in academia are:

- Refusal to take on a task, even if it is reasonable
- Purposefully not completing a task efficiently
- Spreading gossip and rumors
- Going "over the boss's head" and complaining to others in the institution
- "Borrowing" power from outside institutions such as unions in order to exert pressure on a manager (Birks, 2014, p. 1686)
- Bringing in lawyers or other governmental representatives in order to harass victims (Birks, 2014, p. 1686)

- Overt rude behavior and remarks both in person and within social media to both fellow faculty and students
- Hazing new staff
- Being unwelcoming to new staff
- Abuse of power
- Not carrying one's share of the workload
- Isolating, marginalizing, or avoiding a colleague
- Not communicating effectively with other faculty
- Passive-aggressive behavior
- Unreasonable demands
- Feeling threatened by a colleague's qualifications or accomplishments
- Lying about a colleague, slandering
- Withholding information
- Little to no orientation for new faculty or clinical instructors
- Evaluations and feedback based on negative or false information
- Shouting at colleagues, throwing objects
- Lack of support for faculty-approved projects
- "Reporting" to deans on colleagues' work
- Lack of investigation of reported bullying events
- Deans lacking emotional intelligence
- Leadership and colleagues failing to recognize that they are bullies
- Bullying through e-mails—sending threatening or harassing e-mails
- Not communicating critical information
- Making uninformed decisions because faculty staff input was not requested
- Those with tenure acting in whatever way they choose without fear of reprisal

BULLYING *BY* THE STUDENT NURSE

The student may be bullied by various professionals, but nursing faculty and nursing staff are also subjected to inappropriate student behaviors as well. Although the number of students who display bullying behavior is usually small, the incident of students bullying faculty seems to be increasing. The reason why there are nursing students who bully has been a subject of dispute just as the source of bullying among registered nurses has been. Do they become bullies or do they enter nursing school as bullies? Education, bullying recognition strategies, and zero-tolerance policies will help to eliminate the nurse who becomes a bully. However, a student entering school as a bully has implications for faculty.

Schools also grapple with the ethical and moral considerations of graduating a student into the health care system who is unable to communicate effectively or establish healthy relationships with colleagues but who is clinically proficient. Schools of nursing should consider stricter screening methods for students entering nursing programs. Grade-point averages and test scores do little to reveal what type of person he or she is who is a potential student. At present, schools do not screen for the moral and ethical standards of a student, and no formal mechanism has been developed for college-level adults in order to be screened for bullying behaviors prior to school admission. Students should also be screened by educators prior to graduation for not only their clinical proficiency but also their ability to effectively communicate and form professional relationships that include respect for both fellow staff and patients. It should be considered, however, that even the process of screening, unless performed by a third party, could also be used against a student in a faculty to student bullying situation.

Examples of bullying behavior by student nurses exhibited both in class and clinical settings include the following:

- Being late for or leaving class early
- Being inattentive
- Using cell phones and texting during class and clinical
- Being unprepared to care for patients
- Being unprepared for class or skills lab

- Talking during class
- Making rude gestures
- Sleeping during class
- Making rude, disrespectful, sarcastic, and/or inappropriate comments in class and online
- Yelling at faculty or confronting faculty during class or dominating class discussions
- Refusing to answer questions posed to them by faculty during class
- Using class or clinical unit computers for noncourse purposes
- Physically harming or threatening to harm faculty
- Cheating during exams and quizzes and assisting others to do the same
- Demanding makeup quizzes or tests for unauthorized reasons
- Demanding course extensions for unauthorized reasons
- Displaying a sense of entitlement
- Blaming faculty or clinical instructors for deficiencies during clinical
- Disregarding other students

Even though the amount of bullying by students against faculty is small, the faculty is distracted and time is taken away from the other students in order to deal with them. The increased stress of dealing with students may also cause the following:

- Emotional upset
- Decreased self-esteem
- Depression
- Feeling of powerlessness
- Feeling of being criticized
- Loss of high educational ideals
- Leaving the profession
- Physical illness

ADVERSITY BETWEEN EDUCATION AND PRACTICE

Staff nurses often complain when student nurses come to the unit. The reasons for the complaints are varied, depending on the nursing staff. Some of the staff just do not want students on the unit because they feel that the students interfere with patient care, forgetting the learning experiences the students require. However, there are other reasons for adversity between nursing education and staff, including:

- Educators who are not current with practice or who are not aware of unit rules, regulations, policies, and procedures
- Educators who do not communicate or collaborate in a friendly fashion with staff
- Educators who do not work with staff when planning curriculum or skill development needs
- Lack of shared goals between the health care facility and the learning institution
- Preceptors on the unit, assigned by a school of nursing, not being fully engaged in the learning process of the student due to workload and other distractors

Also, nurse educators may feel stressed by having to deal with adversity in the clinical area. The adversity they feel may be caused by the following:

- Shortage of educators
- Educators who feel "out of their element" due to lack of skill or experience
- Facility staff members who are rude, uncivil, and bullying to the faculty's students
- Faculty overwhelmed by workload and doing too much with too little (staff and financially)
- Staff who do not work with educators particularly in skill development experiences
- Lack of resources

Fast Facts in a Nutshell

"Academic nurse leaders play a key role in creating vision statements and norms that reflect an emphasis on civility and respect" (Clark & Springer, 2010, p. 324).

ADDRESSING BULLYING IN NURSING EDUCATION

The implications for tolerating bullying in academia are clear. The actions of nursing faculty and clinical instructors are constantly being viewed by nursing students. Uncivil and bullying behavior can be viewed as the norm and therefore perpetuated. Faculty and clinical instructors must, at all times, model professional behavior. Nurse educators should also:

- Work to create a culture of civility and respect among colleagues
- Provide ongoing education regarding prevention of bullying and incivility
- Hold faculty and clinical instructors accountable for their actions
- Provide mentors and preceptors for faculty, clinical instructors, and new preceptors, ensuring that mentors have been educated regarding bullying and incivility recognition and prevention
- Recognize and acknowledge civility and respect
- Work together to develop policies addressing bullying and incivility among faculty
- Work toward stress reduction
- Seek counseling for work-related or personal stress matters
- Work with student representatives to develop policies that address bullying and incivility acted both toward and from students

Further exploration of these issues appears in Chapter 16, which presents case studies relating to bullying in nursing education.

References

Birks, M. (Ed.). (2014). Turning the tables: The growth of upward bullying in nursing academia. *Journal of Advanced Nursing, 70*(8), 1685–1687.

Clark, C. M., & Springer, P. J. (2010). Academic nurse leaders' role in fostering a culture of civility in nursing education. *Journal of Nursing Education, 49*(6), 319–325.

16

Case Studies: Bullying in Nursing Education

Chapter 15 described the bullying experienced by those in nursing education. This chapter presents three case studies that illustrate common scenarios in which bullying occurs, along with the description of bullying behavior demonstrated, probable cause, victim intervention, potential witness intervention, and critical thinking moment.

After reading this chapter, the reader will be able to:

- List bullying behaviors evident in nursing education
- List interventions for the nurse educator who is bullied
- List witness interventions for the nurse educator who is bullied
- List the probable causes of a student nurse bullying a faculty member
- List the probable causes of faculty bullying fellow faculty
- Identify the critical thinking moments in a bullying incident

CASE STUDY 1

Margo is a preceptor and enjoys when nursing students come to her cardiac unit. She enjoys interacting with them and participating in their education. Most of the time, she finds the students enthusiastic, eager to learn, and willing to assist patients and staff. One particular student, however, troubled Margo. When she interacts with the staff or her instructor, she acts bored. She never asks questions and acts like she would like to be somewhere else. When Margo attempts to show her a new procedure, the student rolls her eyes and sighs. She also snaps at patients and very loudly tells them that she is not there to do certain parts of their care. Margo watches as she interacts with other students and her instructor. The instructor seems to tolerate the behavior as it is never corrected.

Bullying Behavior Demonstrated

- Being inattentive
- Being unprepared to care for patients
- Making rude gestures
- Making rude, disrespectful, sarcastic, or inappropriate comments in class, clinical settings, and online

Probable Cause

- Lack of confidence or a perceived lack of skill or a sense of failure may cause anger and resentment.
- By acting with deflection, the blame for lack of clinical skill is shifted back to the person who caused the negative emotion, allowing students to avoid examining their performance.
- Students may feel that faculty and clinical instructor expectations are unreasonable.
- Students feel powerless and lack autonomy.

Victim Intervention

- See Box 16.1.
- Preceptors need to be given clear evaluation guidelines not only of the students' clinical skills but also of their social skills.
- Student nurses need to be taught that violence, bullying, and verbal abuse are *not* part of nursing.

Witness Intervention

- See Box 16.2.
- Preceptors often fail to effectively deal with a student who exhibits bullying behaviors (poor attitude, improper communication style, lack of respect) because they have not been properly educated on how to precept. They lack the student/new nurse assessment skills and fall back on the fact that they do not want to upset the student instead of administering fair discipline.
- All educators including preceptors should be knowledgeable in the methods to resist bullying and horizontal violence as well as to identify them.
- Educators, in every venue (e.g., classroom, clinical area) must model behavior that includes effective methods for reducing hostility.
- Student nurses must recognize that they as nurses do not provide their caring and compassion just for patients, but for all whom they meet and with whom they work.
- Clinical instructors should receive an in-depth orientation and should have faculty members as a source of support.
- All nursing schools and universities have a responsibility to define bullying and design and implement anti-bullying policies and procedures.
- Nursing faculty must become the gatekeepers, enforcing zero tolerance for bullying at anyone's hands (fellow faculty, clinical instructors, staff nurses, patients, family members, physicians, and classmates).

- Students should be made aware of the psychological effects of bullying and also of coping mechanisms to deal with the stress.

Critical Thinking Moment

- As a staff nurse, have you ever witnessed bullying of a clinical instructor or faculty by a student? If so, how did you handle the situation? Was it effective?
- In the future, if you witness a student bullying a faculty member or fellow staff nurse, how will you handle the situation?
- If you are a clinical instructor or preceptor, how do you approach a student who has been uncivil to a patient?

CASE STUDY 2

Michael was a second-year student at a university. He was older than most of the typical nursing students having served in the U.S. Navy as a medic for several years. He enjoyed learning about caring for patients and enjoyed the interaction of the professors and his fellow nursing students. He did notice, however, that some of the students "talked back" to the professors in an unprofessional manner and this troubled him. He felt that out of respect, the students should keep their concerns to themselves until they were able to speak to the professor one-on-one. One particular student was a real concern. She constantly questioned everything the professor said. After a particularly difficult test, the professor was reviewing the answers with the students. The same student who had caused difficulty in the past began yelling at the professor. Michael had also observed cheating during exams. The students used their cell phones to look up answers to questions. The faculty proctoring the exam did not see this happening or if they did, they thought the students were using the phones' calculators on medication questions.

Bullying Behavior Demonstrated

- Sarcastic remarks during lecture or clinical meetings
- Not paying attention in class or during clinical meetings
- Dominating class discussions or always questioning the professor
- Cheating on exams
- Using cell phones during class or clinical

Probable Cause

- Lack of confidence or a perceived lack of skill or a sense of failure may cause anger and resentment.
- By acting with deflection, the blame for lack of clinical skill is shifted back to the person who caused the negative emotion, allowing students to avoid examining their performance.
- Students may feel that faculty's and clinical instructors' expectations are unreasonable.
- Students feel powerless and lack autonomy.

Victim Intervention

- See Box 16.1.
- Students should be educated (as all nurses should be) in what is bullying and horizontal and lateral violence and its impact on patients.
- Educators often fail to effectively deal with students who exhibit bullying behaviors (poor attitude, improper communication style, lack of respect) because they have not been properly educated in the ways to address the behavior.
- Educators need to be given clear evaluation guidelines not only of the students' clinical skills but of their social skills as well.
- Students must feel safe in reporting bullying to their instructor, faculty, preceptor, and, later on, to a unit manager. They must feel that their complaints are taken seriously and will be acted upon and are held in confidence.

Witness Intervention

- See Box 16.2.
- Allow students to freely express themselves about negative interactions they have encountered and how they dealt with the behavior—this sharing may assist a fellow student and could take place during post-conference time or in an open-classroom discussion.
- Students, in turn, must feel safe in reporting to their instructor, faculty, preceptor, and, later on, to a unit manager. They must feel that their complaints are taken seriously and will be acted upon and are held in confidence.

Critical Thinking Moment

- In the future, if you witness a student bullying a faculty member, how will you handle the situation?

CASE STUDY 3

Ms. Emily Sanchez worked as a clinical instructor at a local community college, the same college where she had attended nursing school some years before. She loved her job and loved working with students. She had received very positive evaluations from her students and, when observed, received glowing reports from her supervisors. The students loved her and were constantly sharing with the other professors how much Ms. Sanchez had helped them. She had worked at the college for some time when a position for adjunct faculty became available. She immediately applied for the position and began requesting letters of recommendation from fellow educators. All of those she asked enthusiastically supported her and wrote letters that were forwarded to the dean. One professor, however, openly refused to write a letter, telling Emily that she would make a "horrible" professor of nursing because she "failed to see the big picture" with regard to educating students. She told Ms. Sanchez that she should work for several more years before she even hoped to become adjunct faculty and that she "had a lot to learn." This was the same professor that Ms. Sanchez had seen sitting in a staff lounge reading a novel while her students were caring for patients unsupervised.

Bullying Behavior Demonstrated

- Overt rude behavior and remarks both in person and within social media to both fellow faculty and students
- Abuse of power
- Passive-aggressive behavior
- Feeling threatened by a colleague's qualifications or accomplishments
- Those with tenure acting in whatever way they choose without fear of reprisal

Probable Cause

- Being a new nurse who may lack confidence
- Being perceived as intelligent, competent, loyal, and accomplished, having integrity, and being dedicated to the unit/facility (Castronovo, Pullizzi, & Evans, 2016, p. 209)
- Thinking outside the box and having new ideas on how things should be—disturbing the "status quo"
- Being perceived by someone at a higher level as a threat to his or her comfortable status
- Receiving a promotion or honor that another nurse feels is not deserved (Dellasega, 2009, p. 54)

Victim Intervention

- Work to create a culture of civility and respect among colleagues.
- Model professional behavior.
- Hold faculty and clinical instructors accountable for their actions.

- Recognize and acknowledge civility and respect.
- Work together to develop policies addressing bullying and incivility among faculty.

Witness Intervention

- Take the complaint of bullying and incivility seriously.
- Let the bully know that what he or she has done has been witnessed.
- Let the bully know that his or her actions are not consistent with the policies of the school.
- Suggest to the victim that there is a support system available. If the witness is not readily aware of the support system, support the victim in finding assistance.

Critical Thinking Moment

- Have you witnessed faculty bullying a fellow colleague? How did you handle the situation?

BOX 16.1 INTERVENTIONS TO RESIST BULLYING IN NURSING EDUCATION

- All educators including preceptors should be knowledgeable in the methods to resist bullying and horizontal violence as well as to identify them.
- Educators must not be seen as tolerating abuse, bullying, or violence—model that nothing but respect will be tolerated from any health care professional, student, patient, or visitor.
- Student nurses must recognize that they as nurses do not provide their caring and compassion just for patients, but for all whom they meet and with whom they work.

(continued)

- All nursing schools and universities have a responsibility to define bullying and design and implement anti-bullying policies and procedures.
- Nursing faculty must become the gatekeepers, enforcing zero tolerance for bullying at anyone's hands (fellow faculty, clinical instructors, staff nurses, patients, family members, physicians, and classmates).

BOX 16.2 WITNESS INTERVENTIONS TO RESIST BULLYING IN NURSING EDUCATION

- Students should be taught whom they need to inform if bullying or violence occurs. The school and health care facility policies and procedures regarding bullying must be reviewed with the student. This includes witnesses to bullying.
- *All* nurses should model professional behavior! What is seen by students is imitated by them. If students experience bullying and the bullying is condoned, they will become bullies and the cycle continues.
- Clinical instructors should be knowledgeable in not only clinical skills but also in how to effectively communicate and interact with students and fellow staff.

References

Castronovo, M. A., Pullizzi, A., & Evans, S. (2016). Nurse bullying: A review and a proposed solution. *Nursing Outlook*, *64*, 208–214.

Dellasega, C. A. (2009). Bullying among nurses. *American Journal of Nursing*, *109*(1), 52–58.

17

Case Studies: Bullying in Nursing Administration

Chapter 8 described the bullying that occurs among nurse leaders and administrators. This chapter presents two case studies that explore three scenarios in which bullying is perpetrated by those in nursing administration, along with the description of bullying behavior demonstrated, probable cause, victim intervention, potential witness intervention, and critical thinking moment.

After reading this chapter, the reader will be able to:

- List the bullying behaviors that may be seen in nursing administration
- List interventions for the nurse who is bullied by a nursing administrator
- List witness interventions
- List the probable causes of a nursing administrator bullying a member of staff
- Identify the critical thinking moment in a bullying incident

CASE STUDY 1

Melissa had a master's degree and was staff development instructor and infection control specialist at a large subacute facility. When she first came to the facility, she developed an orientation and preceptorship program for newly hired nurses modeled after those found in acute care facilities. Prior to this program, new nurses had only several days' orientation with no preceptorship guidance and were then given an assignment of 15 to 20 patients. One of the major concerns of the facility was the amount of turnover of new nurses and poor orientation. Melissa worked very hard to correct the situation and created a model program utilized by other facilities within the health care organization.

Melissa also reviewed the current infection control policies and made sure that they were up-to-date and that the facility was following all state and federal guidelines.

A new director of nursing (DON) was hired to the facility. She was assisted by an LPN and an associate degree RN who had worked as charge nurses in the facility, both of whom had been friendly with Melissa prior to their promotions.

Staff educators in health care facilities often became unofficial liaisons between the nursing staff and the administration. Their offices were "safe places" and what was discussed with them was kept private. Melissa took her position as liaison very seriously and the nursing staff appreciated that they had a caring educator as their advocate. She enjoyed her work and developing new educational programs for the nursing staff. Those in nursing administration, however, did not appreciate either her presence or her work. When she met with the DON and assistant directors of nursing (ADONs) for the weekly meeting to discuss the progress of the nursing orientees, they continued to work on their computers and kept their backs to her, not responding to her questions. If a member of the nursing staff called out, an ADON would pull an inexperienced nurse off orientation and place her on the unit, against Melissa's stated orientation policies. If a nurse did poorly during orientation, the DON would tell Melissa to fire the new employee, despite this not being part of her position as educator. This placed her in a difficult position with the remaining staff who would question their trust of her. Melissa was forced to constantly explain to the DON and ADONs the value of orientation and preceptorship in decreasing staff turnover, increasing skill development, and promoting staff *and* patient satisfaction. They seemed to just care about bodies filling a staffing sheet. Administration did not appreciate the value of staff education and felt that the yearly required educational requirements of fire safety and infection control were enough for the staff. They would often refuse to allow staff to attend any educational offering that Melissa developed including those dealing with life support. They also did not participate in the education offerings themselves, thus not lending support to Melissa. The DON and ADONs would ignore Melissa or laugh behind her back when she was around. She was not included in discussions or social situations. She was openly mocked in front of staff and other administrators.

Melissa would bring issues of infection control to the attention of the DON, who usually ignored the indication for additional education of the staff. One incident included an outbreak of norovirus in the facility. The facility administrator, DON, ADON, and Melissa met to discuss the outbreak and its effects on staffing levels and patient care. Following infection control guidelines, Melissa suggested that staff who were ill remain home, per policy, so as not to infect additional patients or fellow staff. This suggestion was met with derisive laughter and the DON stated that the facility was not going to be short-staffed based on Melissa's suggestion. Because her suggestion was not followed, the virus continued in the facility among the staff and patients.

Bullying Behavior Demonstrated

- Hostility
- Humiliation

- Verbal attacks, taunts, insults, and condescension in language and attitude
- Giving the silent treatment, such as excluding and ignoring
- Withholding support
- Belittling and criticizing, faultfinding and scapegoating
- Ignoring policies and procedures
- Demeaning those who pursue continuing education, and not appreciating experience
- Excluding others from social events outside the workplace

Probable Cause

- Thought of as being intelligent, loyal to the faculty or administration, competent, and honest
- Thinking outside the box and having new ideas on how things should be—disturbing the "status quo"
- Being perceived by someone at a higher level as a threat to his or her comfortable status

Victim Intervention

- See Box 17.1.
- For further discussion of how to resist a bully, refer to Chapter 9.

Witness Intervention

- See Box 17.2.

Critical Thinking Moment

- As a member of nursing administration, have you ever witnessed bullying of a fellow administrator? If so, how did you handle the situation? Was it effective?
- As a member of nursing administration, have you ever witnessed a nursing administrator bullying a member of

staff? If so, how did you handle the situation? Was it effective?

- In the future, if you witness a bullying situation, how will you handle the situation?

CASE STUDY 2

Kathy was an ADON at a long-term care facility. She had many years' experience as a nurse in acute care settings and welcomed the change of pace at a new type of nursing. The DON at the facility was very pleasant and took great pleasure in introducing Kathy to her team. During the interview, Kathy had asked the DON why the position of ADON was vacant, but the DON gave a vague answer and moved on to another subject. Kathy was assigned a preceptor and she reported to work as required.

During the weeks of orientation and into the months that followed, Kathy began to notice that the facility was poorly run and the staff afraid to question the practices of the DON. Kathy herself was unsure how to handle several situations. For example, the DON would disappear for hours at a time without telling Kathy that she had left or where she was going. When a patient expired, Kathy was not allowed to pronounce the patient or to complete the paperwork. The DON was the only nurse allowed to pronounce any patient or to complete and submit the paperwork, even if she was not the nurse who had witnessed the death. At one time, Kathy was called to the unit to complete an assessment on a patient who had fallen. She documented the assessment and because the patient complained of hip pain, she called an ambulance to the facility. The radiology report noted that the patient's hip was broken. Several days later, Kathy was called to the unit by the DON. The DON opened the patient's chart and ripped out the assessment Kathy had completed and shredded it. She told Kathy to never document a patient assessment again. Kathy had followed protocol, but she was too afraid to question why the DON would remove a report from a patient's chart. Another patient fell shortly after this and broke a hip.

As was the policy of the state where this facility was located, it should have been reported to the board of health. When Kathy reminded the DON of this, the DON refused to report the injury, just as she had done in the previous injury.

The DON complained about every worker in the facility, often in front of staff and pushed for them to be fired if she did not like them. She was not an advocate of orientation programs, and new nurses had only 1 to 2 days of orientation prior to being given 20 patients. She ignored the complaints of the unit manager of the Alzheimer's unit. The patients were kept in a windowless lunch room during the day without interaction of staff or family. The unit manager knew that this was not proper protocol and informed the DON. The DON threatened to fire the unit manager if she complained. Breaches in policy and protocol were so frequent and common that Kathy was afraid she would lose her RN license. Narcotics were not locked, dressing supplies were kept in dirty conditions, crash carts were empty or supplies were broken or expired, staffing documentation was altered so that true staffing levels were not revealed, RNs were not allowed to contact physicians if, based on their assessment, the patient needed assistance. The DON did not want to "bother" the physician. Kathy continually addressed the issues she found with the DON but to no avail. One nurse told Kathy that the DON said that Kathy was "lazy" and did not like to work. The DON told staff that Kathy was really not "too smart" and to ignore anything she said or to come to the DON first before doing anything Kathy had requested. If Kathy asked for a day off, even for doctor appointments, it was denied.

Bullying Behavior Demonstrated

- Hostility
- Humiliation
- If in management, not allowing another nurse to be promoted, take sick leave, take holiday time, or get overtime or compensation for work beyond a specific shift

- Verbal attacks, taunts, insults, and condescension in language and attitude
- Threats and intimidation
- Spreading rumors and lies that no one refutes
- Ridiculing and humiliating the target regarding the patient care
- Belittling and criticizing, faultfinding, and scapegoating
- If in management, removing or decreasing responsibilities from the nurse victim
- Ignoring policies and procedures

Probable Cause

- They truly feel their comments regarding the work of others are helpful.
- They may be compensating for feelings of doubt, anxiety, and uncertainty.
- They are unaware of how their actions and verbalizations affect other nurses.
- They try to bond with other nurses through sharing of gossip and rumors—but the result of their behavior is still damaging to others.

Victim Intervention

- See Box 17.1.

Witness Intervention

- See Box 17.2.

Critical Thinking Moment

- As a member of nursing administration, have you ever witnessed bullying of a fellow administrator? If so, how did you handle the situation? Was it effective?
- As a member of nursing administration, have you ever witnessed a nursing administrator bullying a member of

staff? If so, how did you handle the situation? Was it effective?

- In the future, if you witness a bullying situation, how will you handle the situation?
- Have you ever witnessed bullying behavior that jeopardized the safety of a patient? If so, how did you handle the situation? Would you handle it differently now?

BOX 17.1 VICTIM INTERVENTIONS TO RESIST BULLYING IN NURSING ADMINISTRATION

- Depending on the feelings of leadership on bullying and if the bully *is* in leadership, prepare for a long battle.
- Have a positive outlook that all, including the bully, will see—be calm and maintain your sense of humor.
- Always keep in mind the type of bully with whom you are dealing; you must control the situation because in a case against a bully who is a manipulator, by being emotional, you are giving him or her more ammunition to use against you.
- Do not ignore or excuse the behavior.
- Set limits on what you will tolerate from the bully.
- Be aware of unit or facility policies and procedures in dealing with hostile behavior and bullying.
- Try not to be afraid. Fear will cause you to not take action against the behavior.
- Begin by attempting to come to a resolution between you and the bully.
- Be aware that if you speak up and attempt to defend yourself, it may encourage the bully to continue the behavior.

(*continued*)

- Give the action a name, call a bully a bully and what he or she is demonstrating is bullying or uncivil behavior, and get it out in the open.
- Document the date, time, location, and those involved. Give specific details of what occurred including how you attempted to stop the behavior. The fact that patient care is being impacted will be important to management.
- Keep copies of all e-mails and other documentation sent to you by the bully.
- If the charge nurse, nurse manager, or DON is the bully, report the incident to human resources and ask for assistance.
- Ask for help in dealing with the bully. Refer to facility policies as to what help is available for employees dealing with workplace bullying and violence.
- If possible, and if you are not in immediate danger, tell the person who is bullying you how his or her actions are making you feel.
- Speak about bullying at staff meetings—bring it out in the open.
- Speak to human resources (or a similar department) in your facility about how to deal with the situation.
- Note and document whether the person bullying you also bullies others. Be sure that all are documenting as well. More proof of bullying from multiple parties will have more of an impact.
- Be aware of your own behaviors.
- Do not share your documentation with anyone.
- Take care of you! Work stress reduction into your daily schedule.
- Do not take matters into your own hands and retaliate against the perpetrator.
- See professional counseling if needed.

BOX 17.2 WITNESS INTERVENTIONS TO RESIST BULLYING IN NURSING ADMINISTRATION

- Be aware of unit/facility policies and procedures regarding bullying.
- Do not support the bullying actions of others.
- Support the victim by providing witness statements, documentation, and any other actions called for when appropriate, such as in a legal proceeding.
- Do not let an incident of bullying occur in your presence. Act to stop it and/or report it as per unit/facility policy.
- Do not join in on a gossip session, or with a group that is teasing or laughing at another nurse. Refuse to spread gossip.
- Support a fellow nurse who has been the victim of bullying. Provide emotional support, validation, and assistance with documentation.

Bibliography

Alspach, G. (Ed.). (2007). Are our interactions nice or nasty? *Critical Care Nurse, 27*(3), 10–14.

Becher, J., & Visovsky, C. (2012). Horizontal violence in nursing. *MEDSURG Nursing, 21*(4), 210–232.

Bennett, K., & Sawatzky, J. (2013). Building emotional intelligence: A strategy for emerging nurse leaders to reduce workplace bullying. *Nursing Administration, 37*(2), 144–151.

Berry, P., Gillespie, G. L., Gates, D., &Schafer, J. (2012). Novice nurse productivity following workplace bullying. *Journal of Nursing Scholarship, 44*(1), 80–87.

Bronk, K. L. (2016). The Joint Commission launches online resource center to prevent workplace violence in health care. Retrieved from https://www.jointcommission.org/the_joint_commission_launches_online_resource_center_to_prevent_workplace_violence_in_health_care

Brown. T. (2015). ANA: "Zero Tolerance" for workplace violence, bullying. *Medscape Medical News*. Retrieved from http://www.medscape.com/viewarticle/850383

Cantey, S. W. (2013). Recognizing and stopping the destruction of vertical violence. *American Nurse Today, 8*(2), 12–20.

Clark, C. M., & Olender, L. (2011). Fostering civility in nursing education and practice. *Journal of Nursing Administration, 41*(7/8), 324–330.

Clark, C., & Ahten, S. (2011, August 19). Nurses: Resetting the civility conversation. *MedScape Nurses*. Retrieved from http://www.medscape.com/viewarticle/748104

Clark, C. M., & Springer, P. J. (2007). Incivility in nursing education: A descriptive study of definitions and prevalence. *Journal of Nursing Education, 46*(1), 7–14.

Clark, C. M., & Springer, P. J. (2010). Academic nurse leaders' role in fostering a culture of civility in nursing education. *Journal of Nursing Education, 49*(6), 319–325.

D'Ambra, A. M., & Andrews, D. R. (2014). Incivility, retention and new graduated nurses: An integrated review of the literature. *Journal of Nursing Management, 22*, 735–742.

Dellasega, C. A. (2009). Bullying among nurses. *American Journal of Nursing, 109*(1), 52–58.

Dickson, D. (2005). Bullying in the workplace. *Anaesthesia, 60*, 1159–1161. doi:10.1111/j.1365-2044.2005.04465.x

Dumont, C., Meisinger, S., Whitacre, M. J., & Corbin, G. (2012). Horizontal violence survey report. *Nursing, 42*(1), 44–49.

Embree, J. L., & White, A. H. (2010). Concept analysis: Nurse-to-nurse lateral violence. *Nursing Forum, 45*(3), 166–173.

Flateau-Lux, L., & Gravel, T. (2014). Put a stop to bullying new nurses. *Home Healthcare Nurse, 32*(4), 225–229.

Fortuna, D. (2014). Male aggression: Why are men more violent? Retrieved from https://www.psychologytoday.com/blog/homo-aggressivus/201409/male-aggression

Gaffney, D. A., DeMarco, R. F., Hofmeyer, A., Vessey, J. A., & Budin, W. C. (2012). Making things right: Nurses' experience with workplace bullying—A grounded theory. *Nursing Research and Practice, 1*, 1–10.

Goldberg, E., Beitz, J., Wieland, D., & Levine, C. (2013). Social bullying in nursing academia. *Nurse Educator, 38*(5), 191–197.

Griffi, M. (2004). Teaching cognitive rehearsal as a shield for lateral violence: An intervention for newly licensed nurses. Retrieved from http://www.healio.com/nursing/journals/jcen/2004-11-35-6/{d69852b1-a170-4a73-b332-0ce7f17edbd6}/teaching-cognitive-rehearsal-as-a-shield-for-lateral-violence-an-intervention-for-newly-licensed-nurses

Harris, C. (2011). Incivility in nursing. *Nursing Bulletin—Official Publication of the North Carolina Board of Nursing.* Retrieved from http://www.ncbon.com/dcp/i/nursing-education-continuing-education-board-sponsored-bulletin-offerings-incivility-in-nursing

Hinchberger, P. A. (2009). Violence against female student nurses in the workplace. *Nursing Forum, 44*(1), 38–46.

Hutton, S., & Gates, D. (2008). Workplace incivility and productivity losses among direct care staff. *Workplace Health & Safety, 56*(4), 168–175.

Jóhannsdóttir, H., & Ølafsson, R. (2004). Coping with bullying in the workplace: The effect of gender, age and type of bullying. *British Journal of Guidance and Counselling, 32*(3), 319–333. doi:10.1080/03069880410001723549

Johnson, S. L., & Rea, R. E. (2009). Workplace bullying concern for nurse leaders. *Journal of Nursing Administration, 39*(2), 84–90.

Johnston, M., Phanhtharath, P., & Jackson, B. S. (2010). The bullying aspect of workplace violence in nursing. *Journal of Nursing Administration's Healthcare Law, Ethics, and Regulation, 12*(2), 36–42.

LaVan, H., & Martin, W. (2008). Bullying in the U.S. workplace: Normative and process-oriented ethical approaches. *Journal of Business Ethics, 83*(2), 147–165. doi:10.1007/s10551-007-9608-9

Longo, J., & Sherman, R. O. (2007). Leveling horizontal violence. *Nursing Management, 38*(3), 34–37, 50–51.

Luparell, S. (2011). Incivility in nursing: The connection between academia and clinical settings. *Critical Care Nurse, 31*(2), 92–95.

Martin, W. F. (2008). Is your hospital safe? Disruptive behavior and workplace bullying. *Hospital Topics, 86*(3), 21–28.

Moayed, F., Daraiseh, N., Shell, R., & Salem, S. (2006). Workplace bullying: A systematic review of risk factors and outcomes. *Theoretical Issues in Ergonomics Science, 7*(3), 311–327. doi:10.1080/14639220500090604

Rocker, C. F. (2008). Addressing nurse-to-nurse bullying to promote nurse retention. *Online Journal of Issues in Nursing, 13*(3), 1–11.

Rocker, C. F. (2012). Responsibility of a frontline manager regarding staff bullying. *Online Journal of Issues in Nursing, 18*(2). doi:10.3912/OJIN.Vol17No03PPT02

Scott, H., & Gates, D. (2008). Workplace incivility and productivity losses among direct care staff. *Workplace Health & Safety, 56*(4). 168–175.

Seibel, M. (2014). For us or against us? Perceptions of faculty bullying of students during undergraduate nursing education clinical experiences. *Nurse Education in Practice, 14*, 271–274.

Smith, L. M., Andrusyszyn, M. A., & Spence Laschinger, H. K. (2010). Effects of workplace incivility and empowerment on newly graduated nurses' organizational commitment. *Journal of Nursing Management, 18*, 1004–1015.

Staff, S., & Sheridan, D. (2010). Effectiveness of bullying and violence prevention programs: A systematic review. *Workplace Health & Safety, 58*(10), 419–424.

Stutzer, K. (2015). Nurse bullying: Stereotype or reality? What can we do about it? Retrieved from http://www.nurse.com

Thomas, S. (2009). *Junior nursing students' experiences of vertical violence during clinical rotations.* Knoxville: University of Tennessee.

Vessey, J. A. (2011). Bullying, harassment, and horizontal violence in the nursing workforce: The state of the science. *Annual Review of Nursing Research, 28*(1), 133–145.

Wilson, B. L., & Phelps, C. (2013). Horizontal hostility: A threat to patient safety. *Journal of Nursing Administration's Healthcare Law, Ethics and Regulation, 15*(1), 51–57.

Workplace Bullying Institute. (2014). Retrieved from http://www.workplacebullying.org

Yildirim, D. (2009). Bullying among nurses and its effects. *International Nursing Review, 56*, 504–511.

Yildiz, S. (2007). A "new" problem in the workplace: Psychological abuse (bullying). *Journal of Academic Studies, 9*(34), 113–128.

Young, S. (2011). Does nursing school facilitate vertical and horizontal violence? *Tennessee Nurse, 74*(3), 1–2.

Index

academic abuse, 115
academic incivility, 14
adversity between education and practice, 159
American Association of Critical Care Nurses, 5
American Nurses Association (ANA), 1, 4, 30, 43, 76, 84
ANA Code of Ethics, 5, 24, 26
  Code of Ethics provisions, 6–7
ask a lawyer, 110–111

backstabbing nurse, the, 35
bully
  consistent, 95–97
  highly aggressive, 97–99
  typical, 94–99
bullying
  actions, 10
  actions against, 68–71
  adult, 11–12
  break the chain, 72–73
  categories, 13
  children, 11–12
  combating, 93
  coping with, 67–68
  cycle of, 38–39
  effects on individual nurse, 66–67
  girl, 12–13
  health care system, and the, 58–59
  investigation, 86–87
  law, and the, 102–107
  mental preparation, 90–93
  negative effects, 16
  resisting, 89
  response, 89–90
  signs of, 13, 66, 74–75
  terms, 14
  types, 14–16
bullying and the novice nurse, 137
  case studies, 143–151
  effects of, 138
  preceptor role, 139–142
  statistics, 139

bullying and the student nurse, 113
  addressing the situation, 119–122
  bullying of the student nurse, 114–116
  case studies, 125–135
  effects on the student, 118–119
  types of bullying, 116–118
bullying by the student nurse, 156–157
  behavior, 157–158
bullying in nursing administration, case studies, 173–182
bullying in nursing education, 153
  addressing, 160–161
  behavior, 155–156
  case studies, 163–171
  root causes, 154–155

civic environment, 25
clique nurse, the, 35
cycle of bullying, 38–39

empowerment, 88

Green With Envy nurse, the, 35

horizontal hostility, 15–16
horizontal violence, 15–16

Incivility, 17
  academic setting, 18–19
  assessment, 20
  behaviors, 20–22
  defined, 17–18
  different from bullying, 19–20
  effects, 23–24
  intervention, 24–26
  leads to bullying, 22
  stress, 18–19

Joint Commission, 4, 5, 24, 80

leadership standards, 80
leaders take action, 82–86
legal claims, 104–107
liability, theories of, 106

nurse bully, 29, 30
  actions, 30–32
  defined, 30
  patterns, 34–36
  theories, 37–38
  triggers, 32–33
nurse disruptive behavior, 14

PGR nurse, the, 34
physician disruptive behavior, 14
promote civility, 26–27

relational aggression, 15

silent acceptance, 80–82
supernurse, the, 34

terms, bullying, 14–16

verbal abuse, 32
vertical violence, 15

walking wounded nurse, healing the, 75–76
workplace bullying, 15

workplace mistreatment, 15
workplace violence, 43
  defined, 44
  hazard prevention control, 50–52
  management commitment and employee participation, 47–48
  measures to decrease, 46
  OSHA guidelines, 47
  recordkeeping and program evaluation, 53–55
  safety and training, 52–53
  sources, 44–45
  workplace analysis and hazard identification, 48–50
wounded healer, nurse as, 39–40

zero tolerance, 7, 76–77

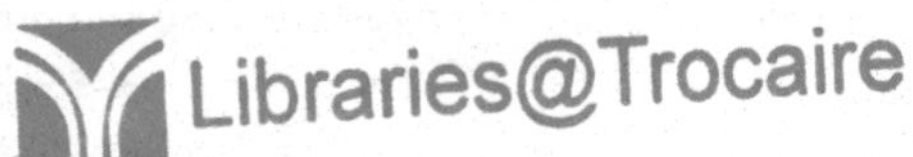